BREAK THE BINGE EATING CYCLE

Stop Self-Sabotage and Improve Your Relationship With Food

Silvana Siskov

Thank you for purchasing
Break the Binge Eating Cycle

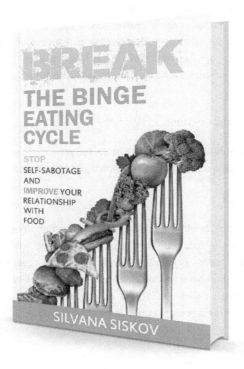

To get the most out of the book, download the free Workbook at bit.ly/binge-eating-workbook.

BREAK THE BINGE EATING CYCLE

www.silvanasiskov.com

Copyright © 2021 SILVANA SISKOV

PAPERBACK ISBN: 978-1-9162424-8-7

Limits of Liability and Disclaimer of Warranty

The author and publisher shall not be liable for your misuse of the enclosed material. This book is strictly for informational and educational purposes only.

Warning Disclaimer

The purpose of this book is to educate and entertain. The author and/or publisher do not guarantee that anyone following these techniques, suggestions, tips, ideas, or strategies will become successful. The author and/or publisher shall have neither liability nor responsibility to anyone with respect to any loss or damage caused, or alleged to be caused, directly or indirectly by the information contained in this book.

Medical Disclaimer

The medical or health information in this book is provided as an information resource only, and is not to be used or relied on for any diagnostic or treatment purposes. This information is not intended to be patient education, does not create any patient-physician relationship, and should not be used as a substitute for professional diagnosis and treatment.

Printed in the United States and the United Kingdom.

Table of Contents

*"Do not let your mind bully your body
into believing it must carry the burden of its
worries."*

Astrid Alauda

Introduction

The world can be a confusing and sometimes difficult place to be.

There is a great deal of stress, anguish, and challenging situations to deal with on a daily basis. Although these things are often balanced by positives. It is sometimes hard to see the wood for the trees when you are in the middle of something that is taking up all your time and thoughts.

When these things happen, how do you deal with difficult emotions?

There is no right or wrong answer, and everyone deals with difficult emotions in their own way. But there is one thing you need to be aware of — destructive methods of coping with hard times can lead you towards very harmful places. I'm not talking about taking drugs, drinking too much alcohol, or smoking to excess; I'm talking about another coping strategy that many of us consistently turn to in order to deal with difficult emotions — binge eating.

Many people tend to overlook this, but binge eating is the most common eating disorder and is a typical way of dealing with stress, anxiety, sadness, or any worry that you struggle to cope with. We often don't see overeating or bingeing as a problem until it becomes a serious issue that negatively affects our lives.

The fact that you have picked up this book tells me that you are interested in learning more about what binge eating is, how to control it, and how to move past it. Great start! However, the road towards overcoming a binge eating disorder, also referred to as BED, is long and winding. But that does not mean it is insurmountable.

This book will give you the answers that you have been searching for to remedy your struggle. It will provide you with clarity and teach you actionable steps that you can take to help overcome the issues you have with binge eating.

Understanding what is happening below the surface is vital if you habitually turn to food as a coping mechanism every time you feel emotionally challenged. Sometimes, it can seem as though the only way to feel better is to reach for unhealthy foods to numb the pain of the problem you are experiencing. If this sounds familiar, you are not alone. Overeating is a common behaviour that many people engage in order to deal with their problems.

As a counsellor, nutritionist, and health coach, I have helped many people with their emotional eating and binge eating behaviour. I know what it feels like; I have seen it with my own eyes. But I have also noticed that it can be overcome with hard work and focus.

It's not easy, and it will not happen overnight. But by taking the time and making an effort, you can live a happy and binge-free life. You can learn to enjoy food in a manner that teaches you about health and moderation, and you can do it all without feeling guilty or ashamed of yourself and your actions.

The reason why you want to stop binge eating and develop a healthy relationship with food is personal to you. Your motivation might be that you want to be healthy, lose weight, or gain control over your eating habits. Whatever it is, this book will help you to understand the deeper reasons behind your binge eating. It will change your mindset towards food and encourage you to change your eating habits. I am not going to promise that all of this can be done overnight — it cannot. Changing your behaviour takes time and effort, but the bottom line is that it CAN be done.

You can gain control over your eating habits and learn to enjoy food healthily and in moderation. And you can learn to deal with difficult emotions more constructively. That is what this book will teach you.

You will learn how to deal with binge eating and eradicate it from your life. You will be able to assess your relationship with food, unearth your coping mechanisms, understand mindful eating, and learn about healthy meal planning. Before starting, however, you need to understand why you reach for food as an emotional crutch in the first place.

Why Should You Listen to Me?

I have supported people in their journeys towards optimum health for many years, and I am passionate about what I do. I have years of training and experience in psychology, counselling, and nutrition. To help you break the cycle of binge eating matters to me. Why? Because making changes to my own diet and lifestyle has proved to be one of the best things I have ever done. It helped me to become healthier and happier, and I want you to feel this way too.

Now, you might be wondering whether this is the book for you. You might also be wondering whether you have a binge eating problem. Maybe you think that binge eating applies only to extreme behaviour, such as raiding the fridge to excess and then feeling shameful about it.

However, binge eating is an umbrella term for a wide range of behaviours.

I will use the term "binge eating disorder" throughout this book, and I will use it as an umbrella term for any behaviour related to binge eating. This might include eating a lot, eating very quickly, eating a considerable amount of food to make yourself feel better, or eating more than you know you should. If you can relate to some or all of these points, the advice I give you in this book will help you regardless of whether your particular situation is a diagnosable binge eating disorder or not.

Binge eating disorder (BED) can be mild, moderate, or severe. It can come and go, or it can be constant. It might be something you do to feel better or to numb your emotions. It is important to know that binge eating does not need to be a life sentence. I sincerely hope that this book will give you a ray of hope and teach you how to deal with your problems healthily and more constructively, rather than searching for relief in eating large amounts of unhealthy foods.

The road towards overcoming binge eating will not be smooth, but it will be worth taking. Each step you take will get you closer to your overall goal. You will not be alone on this journey. I will be with you every step of the way.

Now, are you ready to learn how to overcome your binge eating and discover how to crack the cycle for good?

Let's do it!

Chapter 1

What Exactly is Binge Eating, and What are the Risks?

"A life of discipline is better than a life of regret."

Jim Rohn

The problem with binge eating is that it is such a blurry term. It is often confused with overeating and eating disorders. These eating habits have very different meanings, but they are linked to a certain degree. One can lead towards another if they are left to fester for long enough. Someone who turns to food whenever life gets tough and starts binge eating is at a considerable risk of developing an eating disorder, which can become life-threatening and even fatal in some cases.

This chapter explains what binge eating is versus what it is not. You will learn why it is dangerous and what risk factors are associated with it if left untreated.

There are many serious risks associated with binge eating. Though bingeing is hard to deal with and is potentially dangerous to your health, I can assure you that it is manageable and even treatable over the long-term.

It is possible to stop binge eating, break unhealthy patterns, and replace them with healthier options — trust me when I say this. You can control the binge eating cycle before it starts having a severe impact on your health and life in general.

An important point to remember is that many people struggle with binge eating but do not have a diagnosable binge eating disorder (BED). That does not mean that their problem is not serious or their situation will not lead towards something more severe in the future. It does, however, mean that the advice for breaking the cycle is the same.

So, even if you are not sure if you are in the disorder range, the advice throughout this book will help you examine your motivations for binge eating to whatever degree it affects you and help you break the cycle for good. You will gain clarity about your issues and the ability to manage any potential future problems that could lead you to binge eating again.

Now, let's break it down and define the term.

What is Binge Eating?

We often hear about eating disorders such as anorexia or bulimia, but BED is far more common. The problem is that it flies under the radar to a certain degree and people do not assume that they need help despite struggling with it every single day.

To give you an idea of how prevalent BED is, here are some statistics:

- Around 5 million women and 3 million men in the US struggle with BED[1]

This information shows how common BED is, as well as how serious the problem is. But what exactly is binge eating? What do you do if you regularly binge eat? And how can you know whether you have a binge eating disorder or not?

BED is exactly what the name suggests. It is a psychiatric disorder, and it affects around 2% of the worldwide population. When you binge eat, you eat more food than you should in one go or more food than your stomach can handle at once.

Those suffering from a BED often repeat the process on a regular basis, and it's categorised by the feeling of a lack of control. These recurring episodes can often be triggered by experiencing difficult emotions, from sadness, tiredness, and anxiety, to boredom, loneliness, or feeling unloved. What causes you to binge eat is unique to you, and only you can understand the underlying triggers that create this type of behaviour.

Binge eating is often confused with overeating, but the two are distinctly different.

Overeating is when someone has a little too much to eat at a particular time, for example, when you go out for a meal, and you order a dessert even though you are full. Who skips dessert, right? Overeating occasionally is extremely common, and most people do it. In contrast, binge eating is associated with overeating due to our emotional state and loss of control over our eating. It is less common than overeating but much more serious.

If you overeat because you are on holiday and want to try different dishes from local cuisine, that is standard behaviour in that type of situation. But if you overeat every night because you feel tired, lonely, or bored, that is a vastly different situation, and the intention for doing so is quite different.

After an episode of binge eating, the person often feels guilt or embarrassment, even ashamed of what they have done, and they try to hide it from others. Feeling this way crashes their self-confidence and leaves them with very little fight in them. And when the trigger or problem occurs again, they feel out of control and unable to stop themselves from repeating the cycle.

You might think that this sounds remarkably similar to bulimia, and there are some very close connections, I agree. However, the difference between a BED and bulimia is that someone with bulimia will make themselves sick afterwards, while the person with a binge eating disorder is unlikely to purge their food by vomiting. That does not make BED any less severe or easier to overcome.

For some people, binge eating tends to happen mostly at night. This might be an attempt to keep the binge private, or it could result from struggling to fall asleep, leading the individual towards the fridge. The reasons are personal, but observations of this behaviour initially led BED to be called Night Eating Syndrome.

Albert Standard first discovered it in 1959, but when experts realised that binge eating happens at any time of the day, it was renamed.

For as long as there has been food, binge eating has been around. This is not something new. And even though BED is almost always talked about in the context of modern western diets, many of us don't recognise it as a problem, because the secrecy around the practice means that it is not always noticeable. That does not make it any less damaging than other eating disorders that we know much more about.

The Future Picture — What Binge Eating Looks Like When Left Undiagnosed

You might think that eating too much occasionally would not give you substantial health problems, other than perhaps leading to weight gain, but that is the tip of the iceberg. The key term is "occasionally." When you occasionally eat a little too much, nothing terrible happens, other than perhaps heartburn or a stomach upset. However, a prolonged and undiagnosed BED can lead to the following health complications over time. A few of them are:

- Anxiety
- Depression
- Heart disease
- Obesity
- Diabetes
- Irritable Bowel Syndrome (IBS)
- Sleep issues
- Chronic pain conditions
- High blood pressure
- Fertility issues for women
- Problems in pregnancy
- A risk of PCOS (Polycystic Ovarian Syndrome)

As you can see, an undiagnosed BED is not something to ignore or take lightly. These are all conditions with a range of risk factors of their own. For instance, sleep issues can lead to sleep deprivation, causing problems with focus and concentration. This can also put you at risk of possible mental health issues. High blood pressure associated with BED can drastically affect your risk factors for heart attack, stroke, and cardiovascular disease. Obesity can also cause various health issues, including some types of cancer. The list goes on.

The problem is that even if people are aware of the health issues caused by their binge eating behaviour and appear to know what they are doing to themselves, most will continue with their binge eating cycle.

It is important to keep in mind that even though regular binge eating episodes can be difficult to manage, the truth is that binge eating can be controlled and overcome. However, you must first acknowledge the problem, and from there, you need to make a conscious effort to deal with it. It won't happen overnight, but every small amount of progress is a big win and should be seen as a step forward in the right direction.

So far, we've looked at how binge eating can affect your health, and talked about the various health complications that can arise from more severe levels of BED. However, the effects of BED aren't restricted to physical health; they can also impact your mental health and well-being, whether in terms of social isolation, reduced quality of life, or problems functioning in social or professional situations.

Someone who binge eats will likely do it in private. This can cause issues in relationships, particularly if it becomes a regular pattern of behaviour. The secrecy involved in binge eating can often cause partners to become suspicious and create jealousy or broken trust. When this happens, the associated arguments are likely to push a person to binge eat even more. The vicious cycle will continue, and as a result, you are far less likely to open up about the real issue.

In this section, we talked about the health and social concerns attached to binge eating. By learning about these issues, you have taken the first step towards overcoming your problematic behaviour. As I mentioned before, the road towards overcoming binge eating is not easy, but it is worth taking. By the time you get to the end of this book, you will learn to be kinder to yourself, allowing you to manage your behaviour more easily and, therefore, break the cycle of your binge eating.

Breaking the Cycle

As already discussed, there are significant health risks associated with binge eating. Your body is simply not designed to consume a large amount of food so quickly, and when this process keeps repeating, it can lead to a range of health conditions that can have a tremendous impact on your life.

Binge eating, which can lead to BED, is not done habitually for no reason. With most people, the psychological side of binge eating is quite worrying. They feel as if there is an invisible force pushing them to binge on food, almost as a distraction or a self-punishment. Dealing with problems and difficult emotions through binge eating often means there is an underlying issue causing people to behave that way.

A little later in this book, I will address the possible reasons for binge eating and run through a written exercise to help you start thinking about your triggers and pinpoint the issues causing you to binge. This will take some deep thinking on your part and perhaps even require you to face some challenging situations in your life. However, you cannot move forwards until you have done this, and once you have identified the reason for your binge eating, you can then start taking the necessary steps to overcome the problem.

In many ways, BED is an ever-moving cycle that keeps going around and around until you put a stop to it. If it continues to rotate without any intervention, it will eventually lead to severe health problems that could take you down an extremely negative route. Healthily breaking the cycle means acknowledging the problem and then working slowly and surely to reach your endpoint. It will not happen overnight, so don't become upset or disheartened if you hit a stumbling block or take a step backwards once or twice; the fact that you recognise the issue is progress, and the more you work on it, and the longer you stick with it, the sooner results will come your way.

After acknowledgement comes exploration, and that is what we are going to discuss next.

You will notice that each chapter of this book has a chapter task. That is where you will be given written exercises to complete. I would like to encourage you not to skip any of the tasks as they are designed to help you look at your issues and reasons for binge eating from an angle of self-exploration. Once you understand your behaviour better, you will be empowered to make changes and take actions that will help you break the unhealthy attachment to food and reach a binge-free life.

Chapter Task — Could You be Binge Eating?

This chapter discussed what binge eating is and the behaviours that define it. But even after the definition and examples I have put forward, you may still feel unsure whether you have a binge eating disorder or a habit of overeating that you would like to get control over.

Many people who suffer from BED remain undiagnosed because no one is aware of their problem, not even themselves. Binge eaters are often unaware of whether they have BED or simply reach for a little too much food too frequently. This is why so many people never seek help or receive support to overcome this issue.

To help you find out whether you are indeed a binge eater and suffer from BED, or if you are someone who frequently overeaters, I strongly suggest you complete the exercise in this chapter's task. It is important to be open and honest with your answers. Nobody will read them but you, so you don't need to worry about being judged or criticised by others.

This is a golden opportunity to be open and explore your patterns of behaviour with honesty. Only by doing this can you give yourself the best foundation for building a healthy relationship with food, helping you establish healthy eating patterns and stop binge eating.

Now, I would like you to go to bit.ly/binge-eating-workbook and download the free workbook to help you work through this exercise. The *Binge Eating Workbook* will help you keep everything in one place as every exercise in this book is interconnected. Each exercise is a segment of a wider process towards managing your eating habits.

The questions and exercises that I want you to complete are as follows:

- Write down the last time you remember binge eating.
- Do you do this regularly?
- How frequently do you eat in this way?
- How do you usually feel during binge eating, and how do you feel afterwards? Do you feel guilty or

ashamed? Try and pinpoint the emotion(s) you feel during and after binge eating.

Completing tasks at the end of each chapter will encourage you to take a more in-depth look at your problems and explore the connection between your behaviour and your feelings. How successful you will be in breaking the binge eating cycle comes down to honesty with yourself and understanding the reasons for your bingeing. If you are displaying regular binge eating patterns and attaching your emotions to them, then the chances of you having a BED or a BED-style behaviour are relatively high. Therefore, completing these tasks, which can help you get to the root of your bingeing, is even more important.

I want to point out once again that each person who exhibits binge eating behaviour has different reasons for engaging in this practise, and bingeing on food is a very individualised problem that requires a unique approach. This is why it's vital to go through the exercises at the end of each chapter and answer all the questions that I ask you throughout the book.

All the questions you come across in this book are deeply personal, and your responses will create a bespoke management course for you to follow. You will see that each task links into the next task, and by the time you get to the end of this book, you will have a personalised programme to work through your binge eating issues, triggers, and causes. This will give you valuable information to kick binge eating out of your life for good.

Chapter 2

How to Recognise Your Own Binge Eating Patterns

"Bingeing is such an emotionally frenetic activity that no other concerns can exist in the same space."

Geneen Roth

In the previous chapter, we discussed what binge eating is and looked at its possible effects on your health and relationships. In this chapter, we will explore this further to help you examine your binge eating behaviour and understand the reasons behind it. By doing this, you can start to piece together your behavioural patterns and find ways to address them.

Remember, the advice in this book and the tasks that I ask you to complete are designed to help you dig deeper, explore your patterns and triggers, and ultimately help you overcome binge eating for good. To enjoy a binge-free life, you need to understand the symptoms of binge eating and look at the reasons behind them. They control your decisions and your actions.

Once you start looking at your binge eating habits and symptoms, you will be encouraged to look at how to deal with your emotional struggles and to examine the relationship between the way you feel and how you eat.

Common Symptoms of Binge Eating

Most people think that those who engage in binge eating behaviour regularly tend to be overweight or obese. It makes sense to believe that eating a large amount of food regularly leads to weight gain, but this is not always the case. For that reason, diagnosing BED is more complicated than only looking at someone's weight. Diagnoses are based on cues that are both emotional and behavioural in nature.

Symptoms of binge eating include the following:

- You eat much more quickly than usual
- You eat until you are uncomfortably full
- You eat a lot despite not feeling hungry
- You eat alone because of shame or embarrassment
- You experience feelings of guilt/disgust/depression/ shame

If you satisfy three of these criteria, a doctor will be able to make a diagnosis. However, even if you do not have diagnosable symptoms of binge eating, any signs of unhealthy behaviour around food need to be taken seriously.

I want to encourage you to take advantage of the advice in this book to help steer you away from turning to food as a coping mechanism, and focus on dealing with your psychological or emotional issues in healthy, informed ways. Seeking comfort in food will increase your chances of heading down the road of a binge eating disorder. By paying attention to the warning signs early on and changing your behaviour, you can prevent this.

The severity of BED is based on how often a person binge eats; the more frequent, the more severe the case. But any amount of binge eating is something to take notice of.

There are quite a few potential symptoms associated with binge eating. They include:

- Having a sense of being out of control when it comes to food
- Eating normally when you are around people, but binge when you are alone
- Stockpiling food for later consumption, usually when you are alone
- Often going on diets but not losing weight while you are on them

You must take all these potential signs on board and assess whether they apply to you. Many people who binge eat describe a feeling of compulsion, i.e., they cannot stop themselves. It is almost an irresistible pull and something that's hard to ignore. By realising that what you are doing is in fact binge eating, and by exploring the underlying reasons that trigger this behaviour, you can break that compulsion and learn to control it.

The first two chapters of this book give you the information you need to identify whether binge eating is a problem for you or not. As I mentioned earlier, many people experience this problem but do not realise it. By learning that you have a problem and identifying its source, you give yourself a chance to get on the road to recovery.

It is important to know that from time to time, having an episode of bingeing can be a normal and common human behaviour that will not leave any lasting adverse effects on your health or life. For instance, overeating at Christmas does not mean you have a BED or a related problem. It simply means that you ate too much while enjoying time with your family and friends.

Binge eating behaviour creates problems when it happens frequently, and you experience a lack of control over your actions.

BED is not something any of us was born with. It is developed later in life and can be influenced by social pressure, negative self-image, social media, etc.

There are many reasons why people turn to food and why they binge eat. Each person has their own reasons for doing so.

We are at the point in this book where we need to look at the difference between emotional eating and binge eating. Are these two concepts the same? Let's explore them.

A large number of people turn to food to look for comfort when they are struggling with feelings of sadness, anxiety, stress, tiredness, frustration, boredom, depression, etc. This is called emotional eating. The problem with this type of eating is that the comfort found in food is never long-lasting, and it can be damaging for the person's emotional and psychological well-being. Occasionally, emotional eating can be triggered by happy emotions, but this is a rare occurrence.

If you want to read more about emotional eating and how to deal with it, check out my book *Get Your Sparkle Back: 10 Steps to Weight Loss and Overcoming Emotional Eating.* It is available on Amazon.

The difference between emotional eating and binge eating is that emotional eating happens first and can lead to binge eating. Let me clarify this statement using the following example — your need for a bar of chocolate or a slice of cake might be triggered by your need for comfort and the desire to feel better, less stressed, or to be happier. But when a small amount of your chosen food doesn't satisfy or give you what you were hoping for, bingeing behaviour sometimes occurs. Needing to have more than one bar of chocolate or one slice of cake is very common. Regular repetition of this behaviour can easily lead to a binge eating disorder.

So, as you can see, emotional eating can lead to binge eating, and binge eating can then lead to BED. If this happens frequently, your health could be in danger, your self-image is likely to experience negative effects, and relationships with your loved ones might also suffer.

To help you with the process of overcoming your bingeing, you need to look at how you deal with negative emotions. I suggest you go to the workbook and answer the following questions. They might help you find the answer.

- Are you turning to food when feeling stressed?
- Are you thinking of food when feeling upset?
- Do you often look for comfort in food when life does not treat you well?
- Do you think of food as a life-saver when you are overwhelmed with unpleasant emotions?
- Are there times of the day when you regularly turn to food to seek comfort?

These are the questions to ask yourself, which could help you understand your behavioural patterns better. Only then will you be able to change your eating habits and transform your relationship with food.

How do You Deal with Emotional Upsets?

Most binge eating episodes are caused by people's emotional upsets and unpleasant emotions. In general, humans do not deal with difficult emotions very well; it's far easier to bury our heads in the sand than face up to something that causes us to feel worried, anxious, lonely, or simply out of our comfort zone. We prefer to feel comfortable and safe. This is not what difficult emotions and upsets allow us.

Life is full of ups and downs and navigating your way through your days without ever encountering a difficult situation is simply not possible. It doesn't matter how old you are, whether you're a man or a woman, or where you live; we all face instances of unpredictability, stress, and pressure caused by work, studies, family, society, etc. Even the most confident and self-assured people experience hard times. The difference is, a confident person is more likely to handle difficult emotions in positive ways instead of letting their emotions get the better of them and forcing them to develop patterns of negative coping strategies.

No matter how well you think you deal with life-challenges, there will always be times when you will feel that life has let you down. Turning to food and bingeing will not change the situation and make it better, but can only give you temporary relief that makes you feel worse afterwards. This is not a healthy or constructive way to deal with emotions. It is self-destructive behaviour, which will not help you flourish as a human being.

Drinking too much, excessively spending money, using drugs, smoking too much, or even taking up smoking for the first time are all common coping mechanisms that people adopt to deal with the difficulties they face. Binge eating is just another unhealthy way of seeking out temporary relief from painful and overwhelming emotions.

Whenever you turn to emotional eating or binge eating to deny your feelings or distract your mind, you are not facing your problems or dealing with them healthily.

Bingeing on food can never be a long-term solution or a healthy strategy. Binge eating is a form of addiction that leaves you feeling out of control and can completely take over your life. The difference between addiction and habit is not always clear and compulsive eating is sometimes seen as a bad habit rather than an addiction.

We will look at this subject in greater detail in the next chapter and explore whether binge eating is a habit that you have adopted to cope when life gets tough.

Chapter Task — What are Your Binge Eating Patterns?

Understanding the symptoms of binge eating will help you find out how much of an issue this has been for you.

Not feeling in control of your behaviour is worrying, and to help you with this, I want to present you with a few searching questions, as I did at the end of the previous chapter.

26

Return to the notes you took at the end of chapter one. If you have not downloaded the workbook yet, do it now. This will lead you through the entire process discussed in this book. Go to bit.ly/binge-eating-workbook and download the document to work on it.

Writing things down will help you identify your patterns of behaviour. Seeing words in front of you can bring clarity. By failing to do it, your thoughts will stay in your mind and remain buried with millions of other ideas going through your head every second of every day. Allowing your thoughts to leave your head will help you develop a better understanding of your actions, leading to behavioural change.

The following task will help you examine your binge eating patterns.

Before you begin, I would like you to look at your answers to the previous chapter's task. Use your thought process from there, and transfer it forward to the exercise in this chapter. You will build upon your progress with every chapter task.

Now, answer the following questions:

- From the occasions you identified in the last chapter's task, did you notice any of the symptoms we talked about in this chapter, such as hiding binges from those around you or having a sense of being out of control when it comes to food?

- Do the episodes of binge eating, however frequent, leave you feeling guilty, shameful, or create any other negative emotions within you?
- Scribble down keywords you remember about your feelings during those bingeing episodes and any behaviours you can remember. It might be a little hard to think straight, as the memories might be fuzzy. Binge eating happens fast and without control, but try to remember as much as possible as the keywords you write on the page will create a picture of your situation.

Once you have completed this exercise, look for any patterns or trends that emerge:

- Do you binge eat when you are feeling emotional in general?
- Is there a trigger you can think of?
- Are the feelings you experience always the same?

You are going to build upon these answers in the next chapter.

Chapter 3

Identifying the Causes of Your Binge Eating

"Addictions occur when you seek to fill an emptiness inside you with something outside of you."

Karen Salmansohn

In the last two chapters, we talked about what binge eating is and the symptoms you might recognise if this is a problem you have experienced. Now it's the time to get to the heart of the matter.

This chapter will encourage you to look deeper and get to the bottom of what might be causing you to behave this way. Remember, whether you are concerned that you have BED or would like to curb bingeing behaviours, a crucial part of addressing this is to look for the cause. If you binge eat regularly or semi-regularly, this should be something of a concern, because it demonstrates self-destructive tendencies and an inability to cope with difficult emotions in healthy ways. By examining the reasons for your actions, you can solve the problem before it reaches the point of being a diagnosable BED.

Let's explore the main reasons why people might binge eat.

While we go through the list, keep an open mind and question yourself on whether one of those reasons could link to your own. Identifying your personal causes or triggers is an essential step in this process.

Why Do People Binge Eat?

It's easy to assume that binge eating is all about the food and physical hunger a person feels. This might be news to you, but binge eating has nothing to do with hunger. It's not even about enjoying food.

Binge eating is a psychological response to something else going on inside you, even if you are not aware of what that might be. It's an action that you carry out in response to something that is bothering or hurting you.

It is important to be aware that an episode of binge eating can quickly turn into a cycle that could be hard to break. Let me explain how it works in practice and the steps you're likely to experience during a binge eating episode:

- You turn to food because you feel depressed, stressed, lonely, or anxious about something. This is called your personal cause.

- You might experience a slight feeling of relief when the food touches your lips and you are enjoying the flavours while chewing on it.
- Very soon, however, you do not have the same feeling of satisfaction the way you did after the first few bites, but you carry on eating, hoping for the same good feeling to return and for the bad feelings to pass.
- You binge to the point that it makes you feel physically uncomfortable.
- You experience feelings of guilt and shame, and you feel out of control.
- Then you realise that the depression, stress, anxiety, or whatever you felt before, has not gone away.
- As a result, you feel much worse. So you go back to the one thing which gives you relief, even if it's just for a few seconds or a few minutes before the shame kicks in – and you binge once again.

While drug use and binge eating are not the same things, we can draw some similarities. For instance, we're conditioned to believe that using drugs is wrong and unhealthy, but as with binge eating, drugs provide users with a small amount of respite and make them feel better for a short while. It's an addiction. Every addiction makes us feel better for a short period. That is the reason we keep going back to it. Addiction is a vicious cycle.

With binge eating, you may not crave food or feel you literally "need" it the same way as a drug user needs drugs, but you may feel a compulsion, something you cannot control. It's almost like you're being pulled towards the food, and you cannot stop yourself. You know you will feel good for a few seconds while consuming your chosen type of food even though you are literally punishing yourself. But afterwards, you feel nothing but guilt and shame.

I can assure you that when you binge on food, it is not the food you need. It often begins as a way of trying to control the situation you are in and removing the negative feelings you experience about the situation. You want to deny those feelings. You want to get rid of them. You don't want to feel them. Food is the only thing you can control, and binge eating is the only answer to your problems.

Binge eating is not about loving food too much. You might be craving a particular type of food, but your binge eating behaviour does not show up to satisfy your physical need for hunger. It shows up to cover your emotional need for love, acknowledgement, approval, belonging, etc. Recognising the root of your problem will give you a much greater chance of taking back control and managing your unhealthy eating habits.

Looking at the situation as an outsider, it might be hard to understand the reasons for someone's bingeing. However, when you live with it and go through binge-eating episodes, it makes perfect sense to behave that way. And often, it feels like the only way. This is why the cycle of binge eating is so hard to break.

Everyone who binges has their personal reasons for doing so. We're now going to look at a few common causes. The likelihood of this being your personal go-to is relatively high. However, always be open to exploring other potential reasons for why you opt towards binge eating when you're feeling a certain way.

Let's look at the most common reasons and risk factors that may contribute to binge eating:

- *Gender plays a part* – Women are classified as being more likely to binge eat than men. However, that doesn't mean that men don't binge.
- *There may be a genetic issue at play* – Some people have a genetic sensitivity to dopamine and there is evidence to suggest that this particular condition might be passed down through your family. There is a link between binge eating prevalence and genetics.
- *Weight issues* – Approximately 50% of people with BED are obese. Weight problems can be both cause and result.
- *Feeling unloved* – Therefore, not taking care of your body.
- *Body image* – A negative body image can lead to body dissatisfaction, sometimes resulting in successive phases of dieting, overeating, and ultimately to binge eating disorder.

- *History of binge eating* – People who have a history of binge eating in childhood or adolescence are at risk of continuing the behaviour into adulthood.
- *Emotional trauma* – This can be caused by stressful events in life and drive someone to develop a BED.
- *Regular dieting* – Fad diets often lead to dissatisfaction and a feeling of failure, mainly because they are so impossible to stick to. This can lead someone towards binge eating as a result.
- *History of other psychological problems and conditions* – Around 80% of people diagnosed with a BED also have other psychological issues, including depression, anxiety, PTSD, etc.
- *Struggling with life in general* – Many people who experience life struggles such as stress, relationship issues, inability to meet deadlines at work, financial difficulties, etc., turn to binge eating to cope with their emotional well-being.
- *Habit* – Our lives are controlled by habits that we develop over a long time. Most of them are run on autopilot and it is tough to change habits unless we understand the potential risks they can cause. Until this is understood, the cycle of binge eating is extremely hard to break.

This is not an exhaustive list and your reason for binge eating might not fit into any of these categories. However, it is useful to look at the common causes and see if you can draw any comparisons to your situation.

One of the most common reasons for binge eating is struggling to deal with difficult emotions connected to a stressful event. This could be anything, including a relationship breakdown, sexual, emotional or physical abuse, grief, money worries, loneliness... the list goes on. Someone trying to deal with the emotions associated with any of these types of issues may try to push the feelings away by handling them through binge eating.

It is not uncommon for overeating to lead to binge eating, and then perhaps towards a full-blown eating disorder. To the person suffering from these behaviours, the transition from one to the other appears seamless, which is why bingeing is so often mistaken for overeating. This is partly why it's so easy to develop a BED, and why BED's are so hard to recognise.

The Cause of Self-Sabotaging Behaviour

Binge eating can temporarily soothe your emotions and make your negative feelings "magically" go away. And when life gets tough, that is exactly what you are searching for — something that will take your pain away, something that will make you feel better.

Binge eating provides you with a feeling of relief, even if it's only for a few minutes or a few seconds. You know that this is only a temporary feeling, and you are fully aware of its short-lasting effect, but it feels good. You feel a burst of energy when you satisfy your compulsion to binge, so you keep going back to it.

Binge eating often starts as a method to soothe the pain. Unfortunately, it usually ends with a critical inner voice in your head. This is rarely seen as a positive experience. It's one of the reasons why binge eating is not only damaging to your physical health but also to your emotional state and psychological well-being. The feeling of "I'm not good enough" and other forms of self-criticism often follow a binge eating episode.

You might turn to binge eating to take control of your life, but very quickly, it becomes a habit that controls YOU. Even though you know that this sort of behaviour is damaging, the struggle to break free from it is real. You keep going back to it every time you face a challenge that you can't control.

You might feel guilty about your actions. But you keep going back to it. You might feel ashamed of your behaviour. But you keep repeating it. You might feel depressed about your binge eating. But you cannot stop doing it.

This is self-sabotaging behaviour. It is a type of behaviour that holds you back and prevents you from succeeding and reaching your goal.

It's crucial to look at your reasons for acting this way, and unless you understand the cause, you will struggle to overcome bingeing and will be more likely to repeat the behaviour whenever you face a problem.

Suppose you turn to binge eating every time you feel lonely, depressed, stressed or anxious. These emotions need to be addressed and understood because they are the cause of your binge eating behaviour.

Binge eating is a reaction to your problems rather than a cause. It's a symptom of the underlying issues, not a reason for those issues. Bingeing is a negative reaction you have developed over time to help you cope, but neither the reason nor binge eating defines you. It is simply something you do when things get difficult.

Binge eating can be seen as an addiction, disorder, or a habit. You can see it whichever way you like, but the truth is, it will keep repeating and will be very much present in your life until you understand the leading cause and get familiar with cues that encourage this behaviour.

All damaging behaviours that we display are the symptoms of the problems we have. And each behaviour, whether positive or negative, can be modified. Binge eating is no different.

To understand why you behave a certain way, it is essential to be honest about your situation. Only then can you break the cycle of binge eating and free yourself.

How to Have Self-Compassion

Most of us are familiar with self-criticism and are often unable to accept our own imperfections. We have a habit of not being kind to ourselves, and this often leads to self-sabotaging behaviour.

Many women I work with struggle with self-love and find it extremely hard to accept who they are. As a result, they search for comfort from external sources and turn to drinking, binge eating, over-spending, over-working, or over-exercising. They use these behaviours as a way of suppressing or removing the negative feelings of discomfort.

I have a question for you: What can you do to let go of your lack of empathy towards yourself and develop self-compassion?

Pause for a minute before answering this question. Give yourself time to think. Be honest with yourself. Write it down.

Here are a few ideas that could help you develop self-compassion and break the cycle of self-sabotaging behaviour:

- Notice your self-talk: Is it positive or negative? Does it lift you or push you down?
- Celebrate all your achievements and be proud of them; it doesn't matter how small they are.
- Give kindness to yourself the way you give it to others. You are important too.
- Acknowledge your struggles. It will help you understand yourself better.

- Spend time with yourself and enjoy the moment. You are lucky to have you.

The most important relationship that you will ever have is the one you have with yourself. I encourage you to pay special attention to this relationship and nurture it. Don't overlook the importance of it. It's a stepping stone from which you develop healthy relationships with other people. Recognising the power of self-love and learning to apply it will help you create patterns of behaviour that will serve you well instead of punishing you.

Giving yourself a pat on the back is what you need to do sometimes. It's an empathic reaction to yourself, showing that you matter and are important. Self-care is not only about healthy eating and exercising. It's much more than that. It's about acknowledging your own needs and recognising their value.

Life is full of emotional upsets. We experience them all the time. But it is the way we deal with these upsets that really matter, especially in moments when we're feeling weak and fragile.

Learning to deal with your upsets in a caring way and showing self-compassion will help you to be more empathic towards your needs and, therefore, have a much better relationship with yourself.

Exploring Your Own Binge Eating Cues

To tackle any problem, you need information to work with. For the purpose of this book, this means identifying your own binge eating cues. By understanding your personal cues, you can use this knowledge to prevent a binge from happening.

The causes of bingeing are endless and vary from one person to the next. Therefore, it follows that everyone will have different cues, and it is down to you to identify yours. Our individual needs mean that we need to explore and identify what may push us towards binge eating as a coping mechanism.

Keeping a journal for a few weeks is one way to show your eating patterns. This doesn't mean that you have to write down every single thing you do throughout the day, but it does mean you need to scribble down the important points.

Your journal can be as detailed or as simple as you want it to be. It is a personal tool to help you overcome binge eating, and as such, you can write it in note form or in detail. It's up to you to decide how you want to do it. There are no rights or wrongs, and you don't need to share it with anyone unless you choose to. Consider it your sounding board, your confidante, your record of everything going on in your life, and a way to examine what is going on beneath the surface.

When writing a journal, consider including the following:

- Write down how you feel on each specific day.
- Note anything that triggers an emotional response in you.
- Write down how you reacted.
- If you do binge, write it down.

Keeping a journal will increase your awareness of potential cues such as passing by the vending machine, remembering an event, or smelling a particular food. You probably won't be aware of these cues as you go about your day, because they are so much a part of your routine. By journaling your emotions, your cues should start to rise to the surface, allowing you to become conscious of them for the first time. Once this occurs, you can stop yourself from going down the binge eating route. It's almost like catching yourself in the act, or just before the act, and then making a U-turn and finding a more successful way to deal with your emotions.

This journal will be your personal record that you can use to inform your next move. For that reason, it has to be done in a way that you feel comfortable with. You don't need to include full sentences or paragraphs. You can simply jot down short phrases as you think of them. You can also use your phone, keep a notebook, use an app, whatever works best in your individual circumstances, but make sure that you complete your journal every day to identify your cues and habits. If you stick with it, your journal will expose behavioural patterns that you are probably not even aware of.

You will find an area allocated for your daily journal in the workbook, but as I said already, you can use your phone instead, or a notebook, if you prefer it that way.

Healthy Versus Unhealthy Ways to Deal with Emotional Upsets

The most common reason for binge eating is the inability to cope with difficult emotions and struggling to control your feelings.

In this section, I want to share a few tips to show you how you can deal with your emotional upsets healthily.

Drugs, smoking, binge eating, a chaotic sex life, spending too much money, and drinking too much are unhealthy ways to deal with emotional upsets. They mask the problem and cause you to feel distracted for a short time, therefore giving you a break from feeling the way you do. However, once the temporary high is over, it all comes crashing back in abundance. You also have the emotional, psychological, and physical discomfort to deal with caused by your vice.

As I mentioned before, these unhealthy coping mechanisms are damaging, vicious cycles that many people fall into. However, there are many healthy ways to handle emotional upsets, which are not harmful to your physical health or create shameful feelings afterwards.

They include the following:

- *Exercising* – Exercise causes your body to release feel-good hormones, allowing you to feel better in the moment. This is a natural high that everyone craves, and the good news is that it isn't followed by anything adverse afterwards. Exercise nourishes your mind and body, and it allows you to manage your emotions in much healthier and more caring ways.

- *Talking things through* – Speaking to someone you trust is a great way to deal with difficult emotions. Putting into words how you feel and sharing it with another person allows you to look at your situation differently. Having someone in your life who you can speak to and be open with could be a great support during hard times.

- *Focusing on positive things* – It is relatively easy to fall into a cycle of negativity when you feel down or when things seem to be working against you, but you need to do your very best to make sure you stay positive. The reframing technique is a powerful method to replace negative thoughts with positives. It can gradually help you become more positive and mentally stronger, making handling difficult emotions much more manageable. Another example of positive reframing includes focusing on gratitude. This can be an extremely powerful method to use when you feel like things aren't going your way. Concentrating on the things you have and appreciating all the things you love about yourself and your life is an excellent way of connecting to your values and purpose. Doing this can have a profound impact on your mental and physical health.

- *Practising mindfulness* – Mindfulness is a fantastic way to handle emotions because it makes you more emotionally aware and improves your emotional intelligence. Mindfulness teaches you to live in the moment and avoid thinking backwards and dwelling or worrying about the future. You can apply different methods to become more mindful, but mindfulness meditation is a great place to start. It places the power of your feelings in your hands.

- *Following a to-do list* – Binge eating is often characterised by a feeling of no control. An excellent way to take back some control is to try and be more productive during the day. Write a realistic to-do list and make sure that you get through it every day. Not only will you feel more in control by achieving short-term goals but doing so will boost your confidence at the same time.

These are just a few of the healthy ways to deal with difficult emotions. As you can see, they cost nothing but a little of your time and they can bring significant benefits to your life. Not only will you handle emotions more effectively, but your health will be enhanced as a result. Avoiding harmful coping mechanisms and focusing on positive coping methods is a must-do.

Chapter Task — Can You Identify the Root of Your Behaviour?

The focus of this chapter has been to identify your causes and potential binge eating triggers, and in this chapter task, I will ask you to explore the root of your behaviour a little deeper.

Looking at potential causes is a way of understanding your behaviour. If you can identify the root of the problem, this will help you understand your needs and your actions, therefore, you are more likely to gain control over your binge eating.

The exercise in this chapter task will help you recognise the root of your problem. Use the notes you created in the last two chapter tasks and build upon them. Write your answers in the workbook provided:

- Look back into your past and identify cues that often encouraged you to binge eat. Use your daily journal to help you with this.
- In this chapter, we looked at the most common reasons and risk factors that may contribute to binge eating. Go back to that list and try to recognise those that apply to your situation.

Chapter 4

Stop Dieting (It's Making the Problem Worse)

"When diet is wrong, medicine is of no use. When diet is correct, medicine is of no need."

Ayurvedic Proverb

In the previous chapter, we explored possible reasons for binge eating, and you learned about the various factors contributing to unhealthy relationships with food. We also looked at potential underlying issues that need to be resolved to manage your behaviour better.

However, one of the contributors that you may not have considered is a fad diet. I'm sure you've heard about fad diets or crash diets before. While they might not be the sole reason for your binge eating, they could lead to developing an extremely unhealthy relationship with food.

These types of diets are usually very restrictive and often encourage yo-yo dieting. It is common for your body or mind to start craving the foods that these diets don't allow you to have.

Most fad diets are unhealthy and have very little success among dieters. If you want to follow any diet, you must understand the pros and cons of that particular diet; otherwise, you will likely cause more damage to your body than good.

Any diet that changes your metabolism to an extreme level, through anything other than a healthy lifestyle, can lead you down a very dangerous path with negative consequences for your health and well-being.

These diets will push you towards extreme habits when it comes to food, making you even more likely to overeat or binge.

In this chapter, you will learn why fad diets rarely work, reasons to avoid them, and how they could contribute to your risk of binge eating.

Step Away from the Fad Diet!

Marketing can be very smart, indeed. And the diet industry has exploded over the last decade or so. It is easier than ever for large companies to target us with their weight loss products and services, trying to convince us that spending our hard-earned cash on their miracle diets and supplements, can help us achieve the body we want.

Eating disorders were well-known before social media. But to a large degree, magazines, tv, and the film industry have all played huge roles in contributing to the problem associated with self-image. The ever-increasing numbers of young women suffering from bulimia or anorexia are clear examples of this.

In 2018 alone, the US dieting industry was worth a massive $72.7 billion. These companies do not have your best interests, or your health, at heart. Their focus is on profit. There will always be a tremendous amount of competition within a large industry, which means companies are pushing for more diets to market, more slimming pills to sell, and more weight-loss programmes to offer.

Celebrities often jump on the fad diet bandwagon and speak to their fans on social media about their latest diet's success. This does not help their followers, and they often fail to mention the commission they are earning from the diet company in question for delivering these messages to their fans.

The truth is that fad diets don't equal success over the long-term. The results of any crash diet often lead to short-term success and long-term failure.

For the diet to be classified as "fad", it has to follow some or all of these principles:

- Be extremely restrictive
- Complicated to follow
- Cause the user to weigh, count, and classify their food
- Promises large weight loss over a short period

Fad diets are a marketing ploy to target people who want to lose weight fast. Considering that a significant number of people fall into that category, you can see why these businesses have a vast target audience. Also, weight loss is a hugely sensitive subject for many people. With creative marketing tactics and empty promises, it's easy to hook someone into trying a diet, which unfortunately will probably not serve them at all.

I am aware that many people go from one fad diet to another, hoping to find the miracle diet that could help them lose weight and keep it off. There is a problem, however. These diets are not designed to keep your weight off... if you even manage to lose it in the first place. They're extremely unsustainable, very unhealthy, and quite dangerous too. Most of them focus only on weight loss and don't consider its consequences on people's health.

These diets will never help you achieve the health or weight-loss goals you have in mind. As I mentioned already, fad diets are usually part of the money-making scheme that offers false promises, such as losing 10 kg in 10 days or losing three dress sizes by the end of the week. This is not only unrealistic in most cases, but it could be extremely dangerous to your health.

Why Fad Diets can Lead to Binge Eating?

One of the reasons for fad diets to encourage binge eating is because they limit your food choices. This means you are left feeling hungry or dissatisfied with the amount or type of food you eat. Restriction usually causes cravings to kick in and encourages binge eating behaviour. The feeling of guilt is often present whenever you break a rule and eat food classified as a "do not" on that particular diet. This often creates a toxic cycle leading towards the potential for binge eating.

When you consider yourself to have "failed" a fad diet, the feeling of guilt can be quite disempowering. In addition to having cravings and a strong desire for certain foods, you will no doubt find yourself standing by the fridge or going through kitchen cupboards, gorging yourself to the point of feeling sick. Once this is over, you will not feel satisfied, but disappointed in yourself and guilty about your behaviour.

And the cycle continues.

It is important to understand that you cannot succeed at a fad diet; you can only fail. Even though you are most probably aware of this, every so often you decide to follow one of these diets. They are sold so cleverly; almost everyone has fallen foul of a fad at some point in their lives.

Many studies have suggested[2] that restrictive diets and eating patterns may trigger bouts of binge eating. Once you get into that cycle, it's tough to get out of it without understanding the problem and finding ways to resolve it.

The cravings will be so irresistible that not giving in will be almost impossible, to the point where you will need cast-iron willpower (most people don't have this). When your stomach is growling, and your mind tells you that it wants/needs white bread, sugar, a large pizza, or anything else that the fad diet doesn't allow you to have, you are simply going to give in.

Studies have backed this up, with a sample of women showing that when they restrict certain food groups, the associated cravings drastically increase the risk of overeating[3].

No diet allows overeating; therefore, this is a big issue for dieters. The feeling of guilt that dieters experience each time they fail in their efforts is so common and overwhelming. If you ever followed a fad diet and failed at it, you will be familiar with this feeling. You're left feeling as though you have effectively "fallen off the wagon", and that you have thrown all your hard work away. Disappointment takes over, and you look for comfort in food, promising yourself that you'll start your diet the following Monday again.

Does this sound familiar?

It is important to realise that following a fad diet will not help you in any way. It can only lead to harmful and toxic outcomes. Even if you manage to lose some weight while following a fad diet, you will likely put the weight back on, the moment you reintroduce the foods to your diet that you stopped consuming for a while.

It is disheartening, I know. I witnessed many people losing weight while following a particular diet, but as soon as they stop dieting, all their efforts were ruined overnight. The disappointment kicks in; they lose control and start overeating forbidden foods. Overeating turns into binge eating, and it doesn't take too long for binge eating to become a vicious cycle, which is extremely hard to break.

Cut Out Fads and Focus on Health

Choosing to live a healthy lifestyle and eat the right type of foods is recommended for everyone. Whether you need to or want to lose weight, I strongly suggest you focus on eating for health and avoid following fad diets.

In the next chapter, I will discuss healthy eating and the foods you should try and eat more of, versus the ones you should limit and only enjoy in moderation. But right now, I want to discuss general rules for healthy eating that everyone should follow to a certain degree, whatever your situation is.

I want you to remember that healthy eating, whether you desire to lose weight or be healthy, is entirely possible without restrictive eating while enjoying occasional desserts. Allowing yourself to eat all types of foods in moderation will give you more chance to lose weight, keep it off, and be healthy.

With weight loss, if that is your aim, a slow approach is the most effective, and a sustainable amount of weight loss is around 1-2 lb per week. I understand that people want to get rid of excess weight ASAP, and that is why fad diets are so attractive and immensely popular among dieters. They promise people what they want to hear, which often includes losing all the excess weight extremely quickly, eating whatever they want, and not doing any exercise.

Here is the general rule of thumb for healthy eating. I suggest you follow it as close as you can.

- Don't cut out entire food groups (e.g., don't cut out all fats or carbs) and don't focus on drastically reducing calories either. You need a more moderate and gentle approach.
- Swap unhealthy options for healthier options, such as swapping white rice for brown rice or chips for salad.

- Focus on eating more unprocessed and whole foods. That doesn't mean you can't have a slice of pizza occasionally. The key is moderation.
- Feel free to treat yourself with "unhealthy" options every now and then but keep these to a minimum. Banning these types of foods entirely from your diet only forces you to label things as good or bad, leading to binge eating when you get hold of those "bad" foods. You need to be free to enjoy your food, but I suggest focusing on having more of the healthier things as your main staple.
- Try to pack your diet with fruit and vegetables, healthy fats, and whole grains.
- Don't skip meals or drastically reduce the amount of food you eat. Some diets will advise you to skip breakfast or go long periods without eating, but if you adopted a habit of binge eating, then excluding breakfast from your diet can drastically contribute to cravings. As a result, this will give you a far greater chance of overeating and binge eating. Therefore, I suggest you eat regularly to reduce your desire for unhealthy food. Including three balanced meals and healthy snacks daily will reduce the likelihood of binges.
- I strongly suggest you do meal planning. I am aware that some people are put off the idea of planning their meals because they assume that it doesn't leave any space for spontaneity, and they expect a strict approach to eating, which is what they struggle with.

But meal planning does not have to be this restrictive. It is more of a guide to help you stick to a regular eating schedule and to make sure that a wide range of healthy meals and snacks are on the agenda. This also cuts down on the chances of you becoming too hungry to reach for anything unhealthy, and perhaps binge eat as a result. To give you the best chance at meal planning success, you need to understand what to eat (more on that in the next chapter) and then make sure that you have healthy ingredients stocked in your fridge. I suggest you set aside a day to do your meal planning (you will spend less than 10 minutes on this once you get used to it), and then the next day, go shopping for the ingredients. You might even like to meal prep beforehand and put everything in the freezer, ready to cook.

- You need to watch your portion sizes. Even eating healthy food can be undone by overeating. If you are prone to binge eating, it's a good idea to measure out portion sizes and put the remaining food away to avoid triggering binges.

In chapter seven, I am going to talk in more detail about meal planning and shopping. For now, bear these points in mind going forward into your healthier lifestyle.

Chapter Task — Create an Eating Schedule

This chapter has discussed the evils of fad dieting. I hope you understand the danger of fad diets by now and won't be tempted to try crash dieting again. It is a much better idea to focus on a healthy lifestyle, and by doing so, you can be sure to control and stop your bingeing.

The focus of this chapter's task is on helping you to let go of the idea of resorting to dieting and embracing the concept of health by creating an eating schedule. You will put together your own plan that is realistic and easy to follow without making you feel restricted about your eating. Please note that you will be creating a meal plan in chapter seven, whereas in this task, you are creating an eating schedule.

Now, get the worksheet that you downloaded from bit.ly/binge-eating-workbook. You will find an *Eating Schedule* template there.

How to create an eating schedule and why it is essential:

- A schedule will help you let go of the idea of dieting because you're going to create a plan of your own that you can follow and unlike a fad diet, it will not restrict your eating.
- Create a simple timetable for each day of the week, breaking the day into three meals and two small snacks. If you are using the worksheet that I provided

in the workbook, you don't need to worry about this, as I have already done it for you.

- Decide what time of day you want to have your meals and write these down on the *Eating Schedule* template — it is vital to follow this advice. Aim to eat at roughly the same times each day. This does not have to be set in stone, and you can tweak it and adapt according to circumstances. Crucially, if you know you will be eating at certain times, you are much more likely to stick to your plan, since your personalised schedule will create a routine that you can naturally fall into.
- Use your eating schedule to help you plan specific meals in chapter seven.

Chapter 5

A Healthy Balance: What are You Really Eating?

"It is health that is real wealth and not pieces of gold and silver"

Mahatma Gandhi

In the previous chapter, we discussed the importance of shifting away from dieting and focusing on health in general. Only by focusing on healthy eating, instead of weight-loss dieting, will you be able to change your eating habits and transform your relationship with food. But to do that, you need to know what healthy eating consists of.

The positives of merely focusing on healthy eating and not following any specific diet mean nothing is out of reach, and you are permitting yourself to enjoy a bar of chocolate or a piece of cake occasionally. Not allowing yourself to eat the food you enjoy will increase your chances of overeating and bingeing. It's relatively easy to move from dieting to binge eating, but it is tough to break the cycle once you start it.

Including a healthy diet in your lifestyle means applying long-term thinking. Bingeing on pizza, doughnuts, chocolates, or any kind of food for that matter, is the result of short-term thinking and will give you only a temporary feeling of pleasure. Conversely, eating foods that contain the right amount of macronutrients and micronutrients will look after your body and produce long-term feelings of well-being. Consuming the right foods in the right amounts and adopting a healthy lifestyle is necessary to keep you fit and healthy. These practices are the products of long-term thinking which will provide your body with what it needs.

This chapter will help you assess your current diet and help you put together a healthier lifestyle plan that you feel comfortable with.

In addition to planning your eating schedule, which you did in the previous chapter, it's important to look at the quality of your existing diet and make tweaks to promote good health and satiety — this will make you less likely to binge.

I suggest you go through the following questions before you read on. You will also find these questions in the workbook and I recommend that you jot down your answers. Your response to these questions will help you become more aware of your behaviour towards the food you eat.

- What foods do you eat a lot of?
- How often do you make healthy choices?
- What changes do you need to make?
- Why do you need to make those changes?

There are blank areas in the workbook where you can write down anything that crosses your mind while reading this book. It's a good idea to keep everything in the same place so you can go back to it whenever you need to assess your situation.

This is What a Healthy Diet Looks Like

The word "healthy" is thrown around a lot. And we know that certain things are better for us than others. Still, people are often unsure about what a healthy diet consists of and what changes they need to implement to fully enjoy the benefits of healthy foods and a healthy lifestyle.

A healthy diet is sustainable and enjoyable, and it contains all the nutrients your body and mind need to tick along nicely. A diet needs to be balanced, i.e., it needs to incorporate a little bit of everything required on a daily basis. By doing this, you will drastically reduce the chances of bingeing.

A healthy diet looks like this:

- *Eat variety* – Eating various foods will provide your body with all the vitamins and minerals while ensuring that you don't get bored. I suggest you try recipes that give you a range of flavours. I want to point out that home cooking is always healthier than indulging in takeaways.

- *Ensure you get enough fibre in your diet* – Fibre is essential in your diet, not only because it can prevent you from binge eating, but also because it plays many crucial roles in the body. Fibre is also known to keep you fuller for longer, and therefore it can help you avoid bingeing on food. Foods rich in fibre include fresh fruits and vegetables, whole grains, and legumes. Make sure you consume these foods regularly. It will stop you from snacking when you are not truly hungry and prevent your cravings, which often lead to bingeing.

- *Protein is vital* – Protein keeps you feeling full and therefore controls your appetite. Studies have shown[4] that by increasing your protein intake to 30%, you can lose weight and body fat without realising it. Therefore, make sure to include one healthy source of protein with every meal you have. This includes snacks too. Healthy sources of proteins are lean meat, fish, nuts, seeds, legumes, eggs, hummus, etc.

- *Drink plenty of water throughout the day* – Hydration is vital. Drinking water regularly throughout the day can help you on so many levels. In addition to many health benefits, it can also lead to reduced hunger and cravings. Often, when we think we are hungry, we are thirsty, which means you probably reach for food when you do not need it. Studies have shown[5] that drinking between 375-500 ml of water before a meal reduces your hunger level and makes you feel fuller. Always keeping a water bottle with you and taking small sips regularly will ensure you stay hydrated throughout the day.

Many people assume that healthy eating is bland or somehow lacking in taste, but by mixing up your meals and trying various foods, you will find that healthy eating can indeed be very flavourful. I suggest you get creative with recipes and try new things. It's also a good idea to meal prep to save time if you finish work late. This helps to stop you from reaching for unhealthy options and reduce your chances of bingeing drastically.

My book *Get Healthy on a Tight Schedule* will show you how to eat healthily and lead a healthy lifestyle even if you are a busy person. The book is available on Amazon.

The great thing about healthy eating is that it becomes more than a habit over time. It becomes an addiction, but a very healthy one. I am speaking from experience as I genuinely enjoy eating healthy foods and experiencing their benefits, but this was not always the case. Many of my clients also feel this way. And you can feel this way too. The more you notice how good you feel on the inside, which reflects on the outside, the more you will want to stick to your new healthy practices and keep the benefits coming your way.

A Little of What You Fancy is Fine

The biggest misconception about healthy eating is that you cannot make unhealthy choices. Ever. That means cutting out cookies, pizza, bread, chocolate, alcohol, ice cream, burgers, chips, and sweets. Put simply, it means you are only allowed to eat the food that, while tasty and enjoyable, does not give you the craving kick that fatty or sugary snacks might give you.

There is no need to take such a drastic approach, however.

The only thing you need to remember is the M-word, which stands for moderation. You are allowed to have a bar of chocolate occasionally. You can have a burger sometimes, or a slice of pizza. You must think in terms of moderation, weighing it up and ensuring that you don't go overboard when a snack or any food you enjoy comes your way.

Moderation is key to maintaining a healthy diet, and it's the only thing that will help you stay on track long-term. Cutting out all unhealthy foods from your diet is likely to result in increasing your chances of binge eating once the craving kicks in and you get hold of the desired food.

People often find it hard to resist the foods they love. And when we restrict any food in our diet, it is often the food we end up craving. We are not very good at sticking to restrictions forever. Therefore, I suggest you treat yourself occasionally. This way, you will have more chance of succeeding in your efforts to eat healthily.

When you have your treat, my advice is to eat it slowly to really taste it. Chew it carefully, and don't rush. The more you savour the taste, the more you will enjoy it and be satisfied once it's gone. If you rush it down and don't even taste it, you are more likely to reach for another piece or another slice, and before you know it, you will be overeating and possibly even bingeing. As you have learned, bingeing encourages uncontrollable behaviour and creates a feeling of guilt, which leads to a vicious cycle that you cannot stop easily.

The old saying "a little of what you fancy does you good" is so true, but make sure you stick to "a little" and not "a lot". It is far better to enjoy unhealthy snacks in moderation than to impose heavy restrictions, which will leave you miserable and will likely lead to bingeing. Trust me, you will enjoy what you have so much more if you adopt this approach, and it will teach you a range of lessons. You will learn to enjoy food rather than guzzling it down and not tasting it, appreciating the food you took for granted before. And of course, it will teach you about health overall.

So, throw out the old idea that healthy eating means being super-strict. It does not mean that. It means everything in moderation and living a life that allows you to enjoy the odd unhealthy snack now and again, without it forcing you off track and pushing you towards binge eating once again.

When you allow yourself an occasional treat, you will never feel like you fell off the wagon because you permit yourself to enjoy any food you want — in moderation, of course.

80:20 Rule

Many weight-loss diets are hard to sustain. Either they involve complex calorie counting, or else severe restrictions that leave you prey to cravings.

The 80:20 rule bypasses most of these problems. It is flexible and straightforward to use — but how well does it really work and what exactly is the 80:20 rule?

The 80/20 diet, dating back to the 19th century, states that you will use 20% of your resources 80% of the time, with the other 80% restricted to 20% of the time. This principle has been applied to everything from economics to the clothes we wear.

The 80/20 diet uses this principle a little differently. Quite simply, it advises that you eat healthily 80% of the time and allow yourself less-healthy meals the other 20%.

The idea of the 80/20 diet, which I prefer to call the 80:20 rule, is that knowing you can enjoy unhealthy treats at set times makes it easier to stick to your healthy diet the rest of the week. This method can reduce the risk of developing irresistible cravings. Some people find this very comforting, and it stops them from bingeing on foods.

Many of us struggle to live with restrictions that most diets impose on us, but eating healthily 80% of the time and less healthily the rest of the time is much more manageable.

How you manage the 80/20 is mostly a personal choice, but essentially it means that up to four of your meals a week can be less healthy. Many people save this up for the weekend, but if you want to treat yourself midweek, that is entirely your choice.

What is 80, and what is 20?

So which foods should you be sticking for your healthy eating meals? For the most part, these are the obvious ones, and will typically include:

- Whole grains, such as brown rice or wholemeal flour (especially pasta)
- Fruit and vegetables, which are rich in essential nutrients and a good source of fibre
- Lean proteins, such as lean meat, fish, legumes, or dairy
- Unsaturated fats, such as olive oil and oily fish

Foods to avoid during these meals include simple carbohydrates, trans fats, refined sugars, and alcohol. These can be included in 20% of your diet — but still, only in moderation. A slice of cake would be OK, for instance, but gorging on half a cake could undo your good work.

Does the 80:20 rule work?

Many people have great success following the 80:20 rule, especially if they have a history of unhealthy eating or bingeing. Besides its effectiveness at reducing cravings, the meals you eat during the 80% help form good habits. Also, it is the flexibility of this approach that helps people the most. When you allow yourself to enjoy foods on the "naughty" list, it does not put pressure on you, and it permits you to eat whatever you fancy without breaking rules.

However, I cannot emphasise the importance of controlling your portions on both sides enough — 80% and 20%. Additionally, don't forget that any healthy diet must go hand in hand with an exercise regime. Ignoring either of these is likely to sabotage your efforts.

As long as you use it wisely, the 80:20 rule can provide an excellent tool for staying on track. And if losing a few pounds off your belly is your goal, following this rule is a perfect way to lose weight and learn to eat healthily.

Food Diaries and Why they are Super-Useful

I have already mentioned keeping a journal of your binge eating — how you feel before, during, and after. A food diary is very similar to this and will give you a lot more control over your diet and emotions and, therefore, over your binge eating.

A food diary does not have to be cumbersome. You do not have to fill it out every time you eat something, although this might help in the early stages so that you don't forget to enter anything. Once you are in the habit of paying more attention to the meals and snacks you consume, you can leave writing them down until the end of the day. Both options work equally well and can help you achieve the desired outcome, allowing you to keep track of your eating.

You may wonder why this is so important. There are many reasons for keeping track of your food. Journalling keeps you accountable. It helps you move towards healthy changes. And it highlights any areas that need attention.

A food diary will give you an idea of the changes you need to make, and from there, you can start planning your new and healthier lifestyle.

Your food diary should include your main meals and snacks and the amount of water you drink. You should also track your mood. What you eat will have a significant impact on your mood and vice versa. Therefore, recording your mood will help you make the changes you need to create a healthier diet overall. And at the same time, it will help you to address your binge eating problems.

Many apps can help you track your food intake. One of them is called MyFitnessPal. This is a free app that can help you track your diet and exercise. Alternatively, it's ok to use a pen and paper. For your convenience, I included a *Food and Mood Diary Template* in the workbook.

As with everything else, make sure you choose the option that suits you best — you are more likely to stick to it.

After a few days of recording your food and drink intake, you will likely start to fall into a pattern with your food diary and start enjoying it after a while. Looking back over what you have eaten if you have managed to make healthy choices, will give you a confidence boost and a sense of satisfaction. And if you have perhaps eaten a little too much unhealthy food, you can vow to change things the following day and keep your healthy streak going. It almost becomes like a competition with yourself, but a beneficial and healthy one when done in the right way.

Focusing on health is never a bad thing. Not only is it necessary for maintaining a healthy weight and preventing the development of some chronic diseases, but adopting a healthier lifestyle can make you feel good, and it will show on the outside too. Your skin will glow, your eyes will sparkle, you will feel good from the inside and look good from the outside.

Health is a total mind, body, and soul package, and in the next chapter, we are going to look at how to create an environment that works for you rather than against you.

Chapter Task — Start a Food Diary

This chapter aimed to show you that healthy eating can be fun and that you don't need to drastically cut out certain foods from your diet. And if your goal is to lose weight, it is probably a better idea to focus on becoming healthier rather than eating for weight loss. The rest will then fall into place.

In the last section, I talked about keeping a food diary. This is a great way to help you get on track when making healthier choices. With that in mind, this chapter's task is to create your food diary and start tracking what you eat and your general food-related habits.

To help you start with your daily tracking, here are a few tips to follow:

- You will find the *Food and Mood Diary* in the workbook that you have hopefully downloaded by now. If you are using a manual journal such as a notebook or a piece of paper, separate a page into columns and rows to enter the details about food, drink, and mood.
- Begin by tracking your current eating habits before making any changes. Do this for a week or two, and then look over your records — note how you felt on particular days and look for patterns — e.g., perhaps you felt tired on days when you had eaten wheat with every meal — this will tell you to vary up your carbohydrates more.

- When you write down your meals and drinks, use a uniform measurement, e.g., cups, ounces, etc. If you had chips, write down how many you had, and if you ate chocolate, how many squares you ate, etc.
- Continue keeping a food diary but begin to make healthy changes according to your mood, and consider if anything is missing from your diet. Be sure to prioritise fibre and protein to promote feelings of fullness.
- A food diary will keep you accountable to yourself, promote good health, and help you stick to your plan.
- If you binge — record everything you ate during your binge and how you felt before, during, and after. By doing this, you can look back and identify causes, which will help you identify your potential triggers and find a solution.
- Remember — no one will see this but you.
- Doing this will help you face the problem. Don't pretend it does not exist — instead, recognise that it happened and try to understand the reason.
- Writing down the details will also help you recognise trigger foods.

I want to repeat this once again — keeping a food and mood diary to track what you are eating and how you feel will help you keep yourself accountable and encourage you to make healthy changes.

Chapter 6

Is Your Kitchen on Your Side? It's Time For a Clear Out

"If you keep good food in your fridge, you will eat good food."

Errick McAdams

The way your kitchen is laid out and what is inside your fridge and kitchen cupboards can help you or hinder you. The way you display and store food can draw your attention to unhealthy options and tempt you towards eating them when you're trying to be healthy and perhaps bingeing on them when you're not feeling so great and are struggling to deal with your emotions.

With that in mind, clearing out your kitchen is an excellent way to reduce temptation and cut out triggers that could set you on the path towards bingeing. Also, having more healthy food options means that if you feel peckish and want to grab a snack, you are far more likely to opt for something more nutritious than foods high in sugar and fat.

Let's be honest — if you are at home and feeling a bit hungry, and you know you have a cake in the fridge, you are quite likely to choose the cake over a piece of fruit. However, if the cake is not there, you don't have a choice but to reach for a healthier option instead.

Retraining your mind to go for healthy foods rather than unhealthy ones takes time. And to avoid pitfalls, which can and do happen, you need to clear out your kitchen of anything which could cause a significant temptation.

In this chapter, we will look at food storage and the contents of your kitchen and how these things might contribute to your binge triggers. You will also learn the best way to arrange your kitchen for a healthier lifestyle.

It's Time to Clear Out the Kitchen!

Did you know that cleaning out your kitchen can be quite cathartic? Many people feel unhappy and unproductive in a home full of clutter. Any type of decluttering has a very satisfying feel to it. It can help you focus and boost your happiness levels, so an overall declutter is not a bad plan at all.

Let's focus on the kitchen, to begin with.

Your kitchen will likely contain trigger foods, so these are the first things that need to go. You will know what your potential triggers are from your journal and your food diary.

Having those triggers in the kitchen makes it more likely for you to binge and continue the cycle of guilt, followed by more bingeing and a sense of no control.

This is one of the reasons why keeping a food diary can be so beneficial. It can help you discover your triggers. If you found out that crisps are a trigger for you, you can choose not to have them in your kitchen or anywhere in your home and decide to buy a packet only occasionally. Of course, that does not mean that you can never eat crisps, but not having them in your home makes it harder for you to binge on them.

Having your triggers far from your reach makes it less likely that you'll go out of your way to get them as this would require you to get dressed, get in the car, drive to the store, purchase the groceries, and drive back home. Some people might do this, but for the majority, not having unhealthy foods at home means they are less likely to eat them.

If you decide to keep your trigger foods at home and this results in a binge, it goes without saying that you would need to enter this into your food diary. Writing everything in the *Food and Mood Diary* will hold you accountable and stop you from bingeing on treats and going against the idea of moderation. Having a good look at your diary at the end of each week and checking how many treats you had and when will enable you to work out whether you need to cut back further or if you have successfully maintained a balance between health and moderation.

Things to Throw Out and Things to Keep

Your diary will identify your trigger foods. You will then need to remove them from your kitchen. If you choose not to give up on these foods, that is perfectly fine, but try not to buy them with your weekly shopping. If you want to eat your trigger foods, then go to the shop and purchase them separately. This might prevent you from buying them in the first place.

Next, you need to learn the difference between healthy foods and unhealthy ones. Any sugary foods should be thrown away as they are incredibly harmful to your health and well-being. The problem with sugary foods is that the more you eat them, the more you want them. Sugar can affect your brain similarly to the way drugs do. Therefore, you can easily become addicted to sugar, and this can lead to binge eating.

Removing the trigger foods from your home will decrease the chances of reaching for them in difficult situations. Clearing out trigger foods from your fridge and the kitchen cupboards will clear things out in more ways than one.

Once you have cleared out your kitchen from unhealthy food options, you should stock up on healthy food choices. When you are shopping, head to the fresh groceries aisle and stock up on fresh fruit and vegetables. Your shopping list should also include a variety of nuts, seeds and whole grains. These will be the staples in your new kitchen, and I suggest you include them in your healthy meals.

Make sure that you always have healthy snacks to hand. An example of a healthy snack is a sliced-up apple with a little bit of peanut butter on top. This is a delicious snack that can give you that sweet and crunchy element you might crave at times.

Having healthy snacks such as these means that you are less likely to turn to emotional eating and bingeing.

Also, remember that beverages are included in the healthy versus unhealthy subject too. Make sure you have plenty of water on hand. All you need to do is grab a glass of water with a squeeze of fresh lemon and lime inside for an instant refresher and total hydration. As I mentioned earlier, sometimes when you think you are hungry, you are just thirsty, so always try a glass of water beforehand and see if that takes away your need for a snack.

Any carbonated drinks need to go. This includes the diet versions of fizzy drinks because they are full of artificial sweeteners and other preservatives that could be quite harmful to your health. Stick to herbal teas and water, and you are good to go.

By getting rid of any triggers and loading up your fridge with healthier options, you are setting the foundation for your new lifestyle and cutting down on the chances of bingeing in the process.

How to Arrange Your Kitchen

If you want to start eating less and stop bingeing, I strongly suggest you rearrange your kitchen. The display in your kitchen plays a big part in determining what type of foods you will have and how much you will eat.

To organise your kitchen, I suggest you do the following:

- *Remove cardboard boxes and put the food in clear containers* – It's easier to overeat when you can't see how quickly food is going down.
- *Keep food out of sight* – Keep your clear containers out of sight. It's easier to resist food you cannot see.
- *Do not mix cutlery and plates with your food storage cupboards* – Keeping them separate will give you a greater chance of success. It will minimise the temptation of reaching for foods as you open a cupboard to look for a plate.
- *Clear out kitchen items you do not use (this includes your trigger foods)* – We are more likely to reach for unhealthy snacks when we feel stressed. A cluttered kitchen creates a cluttered mind, leading to stress and making you less inclined to cook from scratch.
- *Buy food in smaller packages* – Instead of buying family size packaged foods, choose smaller

packaging. It can help you not to overeat. It will probably be more expensive, but buying a bigger size and then bingeing on it, will not save you money. You are likely to spend more money by doing this.

- *Keep a bowl of fruit or other healthy foods visible and easy to reach* – When hunger strikes, you are likely to grab a piece of fruit or another healthy option because it's there, instead of searching for something unhealthy.

Declutter your kitchen, and you will be less stressed — you will have more space, and you will be healthier for it.

Chapter Task — Clear Out Your Kitchen

This chapter discussed why you need to declutter your kitchen and start organising it with health in mind. Your task is to act on the advice given in this chapter and clear out your kitchen.

This is how to do it:

- Consult your food diary and note what your trigger foods are.
- Remove all trigger foods and unhealthy processed snacks (remember — this does not mean you can never eat them — you are just not going to stock them at home).
- Go shopping and stock up on healthy snacks.

- Transfer food into clear containers and keep them out of sight.
- Remove food from countertops.
- Clear away unwanted clutter.
- Stick your eating schedule to the fridge.

Getting rid of any clutter in your kitchen will create a stress-free, healthy eating zone!

Chapter 7

Take Back Control: Dieting is not Your Friend, But Planning is

"Love yourself enough to live a healthy lifestyle."

Jules Robson

If you look back at chapter four, you will remember that I briefly mentioned meal planning.

Meal planning is a useful and positive habit to have. Therefore, I am going to talk about it in more detail in this chapter. I want to show you why meal planning is a good idea, how to begin, and the do's and don'ts. Following the advice I give you, you will be well equipped to start creating your own healthy meal plan.

Meal planning often makes people yawn because not many people understand the benefits. Also, planning meals can seem daunting. This is because planning out the things you're going to eat when you have never really had control over your eating before can seem like a mountain to climb. Therefore, creating an achievable plan and something you will enjoy is crucial.

The word "planning" can often sound misleading. It makes it sound like a set of firm guidelines that you need to follow, almost like rules. While you should try and stick to your plan as much as possible, it doesn't mean that you can't move things around and tweak them, or that you can't have a treat when you want one. Remember, moderation is key.

Meal Planning doesn't have to be Boring

The word "planning" brings to mind boredom for many people.

I understand that you want to have a certain amount of spontaneity with your food and that if you fancy something in the moment, you want to have the freedom to enjoy it.

One of the common misconceptions people have is that they need to stick to the plan rigidly. Many people don't understand that meal planning does not need to take freedom away from you. It is a guideline, and as long as any tweaks you make do not cause your daily food intake to go from healthy to unhealthy, there is no problem with moving things around a little.

There are many reasons why meal planning is very instrumental in developing healthy eating patterns. Apart from helping you gain control over your food and avoid binge eating, it also saves you time and money. Being organised is an underrated skill!

If you think about how much it costs to order a takeaway because you got home late from work and are too tired to cook, planning your meals can save you lots of money. To save time, you can take food out of the freezer to defrost in advance of cooking or make sure that veggies and other ingredients are chopped and ready beforehand. Home-cooked meals are often healthier alternatives to takeaways, which are usually loaded with extra salt, preservatives and high in fats, which negatively affect our health.

Being organised means that you are not going to be as tempted to call your local delivery number. This does not mean you can never have any delivery food such as Chinese, Indian, or pizza, but you are less likely to do so. Occasionally treating yourself is fine, but having regular treats could damage your health.

If you have had a busy and stressful day or feel too tired to cook, this can create a significant risk of reaching for foods high in fats and sugar and bingeing on them. Meal planning can help avoid all of this while making you feel more in control of your bingeing.

Planning your meals also makes it much easier to stick to your eating schedule of three balanced meals and two snacks. If you can see it written down, you are more likely to stick to it.

If you love to write lists, you might welcome this approach as it's designed to help you eat more healthily. You are likely to gain more control over your eating patterns as a result, and after sticking to the meal plan for a day, the following day, and the day after that, it can create a sense of achievement.

This does not mean you will never have a day that doesn't go according to plan, but the idea is to be as near to ideal as possible, without forcing yourself to be perfect. Do you remember the section in this book about the 80:20 rule? That's what I'm talking about — eat right 80% of the time, and permit yourself to eat less healthy for the remaining 20%, and you will be just fine.

How to Begin Meal Planning

Doing your weekly meal plan might put you out of your comfort zone, but by starting slowly and making sure that all the basics are covered, you will begin to feel more comfortable doing this task.

Each of your meals should contain:

- Protein
- Complex carbohydrates
- Vegetables

You can do this in quarters, mentally dividing your plate with one quarter reserved for protein, a quarter for carbohydrates, and two quarters (half the plate) left for fresh vegetables. That will give you all the nutrients and energy you need for good health and well-being. It will also ensure that you stay fuller for longer due to protein and slow-release fibre. It is also important to add fatty foods to your meals, including coconut oil, avocado, or oily fish.

This is what the balanced eating plate looks like when divided into three parts:

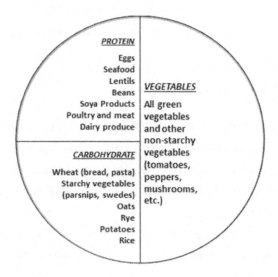

If you follow these guidelines, you will have a balanced diet. A healthy diet will control your blood sugar levels and prevent you from craving sugar and foods rich in simple carbohydrates. Disrupted blood sugar levels can cause poor sleep, depression, anxiety, low energy, brain fog, and sugar cravings. These are all leading factors to binge eating. A healthy and balanced diet will make sure your energy level is stable and your brain is sharp.

It a good idea to mix up your meals and do not stick to the same few dishes all the time. Eating the same meals continuously will not provide your body with the variety of nutrients needed for healthy functioning and growth, and it could cause boredom with the food you eat. This might push you back to your usual routine — eating unhealthy foods and bingeing. Novelty provides us with different options, makes us curious, and encourages us to discover new things.

When planning your meals, make a plan that you can stick to, which will help you maintain control.

Try different recipes and mix things up a little. You might find that you like ingredients that you never tried before. For instance, maybe you have never tried sweet potato, which is very healthy. Try it once and see if you like it. If you don't enjoy it, that's fine; you do not need to have it. Healthy eating is not about forcing yourself to eat foods you don't like just because they fall within the healthy brackets; it's about discovering what healthy foods you like so you can make meals you enjoy and be healthy at the same time.

My advice is to focus on becoming healthier week upon week.

Do's and Don'ts of Meal Planning

Meal planning is not an exact science, but to make it work well, there are some do's and don'ts you should adhere to. These are not particularly difficult, and again, meal planning does not involve a clipboard and a strict set of rules. It's there to give you control, save you time, and allow you to stick to a healthy lifestyle that provides you with variety, balance, and a far lower chance of resorting to bingeing.

The Do's of Meal Planning

- *Plan your meals each week* – Choose a day that suits you best when you have time to create your plan and look for different recipes online or in recipe books. Rushing through it will not give you the most delicious week ahead.
- *Write a shopping list as you go through your plan* – This will ensure you only buy what you need for your meals and avoid impulse purchases of unhealthy snacks that could lead you towards bingeing.
- *Mix things up* – Do not have just a few meals on rotation throughout the week; be sure to look for new and exciting recipes and try not to revisit a meal within one week.
- *Stick to more simple meals during your working week* – You are more likely to stick to your plan if you do this.
- *Consider meal prep for your busier days* – If you have more time at the weekends, you can make your

87

meals ahead (the ones that allow you to do this), batch them, and freeze them. This might not be an option with all your meals, but if you were thinking about making a stew, for instance, you can cook it and then freeze it. The same goes for things like bolognese sauce. Advanced meal prep saves you time and makes it easier for you to enjoy delicious meals during the week when you might be too busy to cook from scratch.

The Don'ts of Meal Planning

- *Create your meal plan when you are hungry* – Creating a meal plan when you are hungry could turn out to be a trigger for bingeing. Make sure you have eaten a meal beforehand and you are not feeling peckish. The best time for meal planning for most of my clients is straight after dinner.
- *Feel there is no "wiggle" room* – If you really want to move a meal around, you can do so. Do not feel that meal planning is super-restrictive. Thinking that way could lead you towards the familiar feeling of being out of control. All you need to remember is that if you move a meal to another day and swap things around, ensure it is within the guidelines of what it needs to contain, such as protein, fibre, and healthy fats.
- *Go shopping when you are hungry* – Huge mistake! You will end up loading your trolley with all sorts of things you don't need and you will more than likely

binge when you return home. Make sure you are full before you go shopping. If you feel peckish while shopping, have some fruit slices in your bag or a handful of nuts to munch on.

- *Be super ambitious* – Make sure your plan is easily achievable, otherwise, you will burn yourself out trying to hit your marks every day, and you will throw in the towel by midweek. This sense of failure could be enough to kickstart your bingeing once more.

Chapter Task — Create a Weekly Meal Plan

Meal planning doesn't have to be complicated or tedious. It can be quite good fun, and it will certainly give you back the control you feel you've been lacking. It is also the ideal way to keep you on track and stop you from falling into old patterns.

Your task for this chapter is to create your own meal plan for your first week. You will find a weekly *Meal Planner* and a *Grocery List* template for this task in the workbook.

- Plan meals for a week, including three meals and two small snacks a day, balancing them according to the guidelines I have given you.
- No food is off-limits, but each meal should include protein, carbohydrates and healthy fats.
- Try to include fresh produce in each meal.

- Aim for most of your foods to be whole and unprocessed, but don't forbid yourself treats.
- Aim for a variety of foods and meals throughout the week.
- Write a shopping list to match your meal plan.

Chapter 8

Leaping into Success: Are You Getting Enough Exercise?

"Good things come to those who sweat."

Anonymous

How often do you hear about how important it is to do 10,000 steps a day and move your body more? Maybe hearing it makes you roll your eyes, but when you understand the benefits of exercise to your health and well-being, you will want to pay more attention to it.

To live a healthy lifestyle, you need to eat a balanced diet, focus on getting enough sleep, and be physically active. It's a recipe that needs all the ingredients in order to work.

In this chapter, I will talk in more detail about the benefits of exercise generally and how it ties into helping you battle your binge eating habits. You will be encouraged to get started with moving your body a little more and finding an exercise type that you enjoy. Yes, exercise can and should be fun!

Boost Your Health with Exercise

Heart health is vitally important. When you have a healthy and robust heart, everything else falls into place. A good diet helps keep your heart strong and healthy by providing it with nutrients and oxygen for optimal health. However, exercise plays a vital role in this process. By combining a healthy diet and regular exercise, you strengthen what is arguably the most crucial organ in your body.

And it is not only your heart that benefits from regular exercise; every major organ in your body receives the benefits too. Your lungs get stronger, and their capacity increases, your immune system improves, your brain becomes sharper and more focused, and your mental health is also likely to improve.

Very often, good health and regular exercise go hand in hand. The good news is that incorporating exercise into your life can be very easy.

While it is a good idea to think about doing a particular activity, e.g., swimming, running, playing a team sport, or going to the gym, small changes can also make a big difference. This means you can get a good workout by getting off the bus a couple of stops early and walking the rest of the way, leaving the car at home and walking instead, taking the steps instead of the lift, and standing up for a portion of the day, rather than always sitting down.

Small changes really can make a massive difference to your health.

Pause for a moment…. and think about how much and how often you currently exercise.

My advice is to move your body every day. The more you move, the more you will benefit from it.

Some people exercise excessively as a coping mechanism. If you are one of those people, it is crucial to recognise that you are using exercise as a distraction and possibly pushing your body too much. Learn to embrace exercise as a welcome part of your life, something you enjoy and brings you pleasure. Don't view it as a distraction from your problems. Exercising should be a part of a healthy lifestyle that allows you to overcome issues and not worsen them.

Did you know that aside from contributing to a healthier lifestyle, exercise can help avoid bingeing?

Numerous studies have backed this up[6] and showed that regular exercise could reduce the frequency of binge eating up to 81% across the period of one week. Studies also suggest that cognitive behavioural therapy (CBT) could be more effective for binge eating reduction when exercise is done alongside it[7].

Overall, exercise gives you a far better chance of kicking binge eating out of your life for good while strengthening your physical and mental health at the same time.

The Huge Benefits of Regular Exercise

Many people are aware of the importance of exercising and moving their bodies, but they are not aware of all the benefits. I will mention some of them here:

- *Mood enhancement* – Exercise can boost your mood, decrease stress, and reduce anxiety. The endorphins released during exercise help distract your mind from stress and worries and, therefore, put everything into perspective. This can significantly help people with a habit of regular binge eating. Feeling more upbeat and positive will reduce your need to binge eat.
- *Better sleep and regulate appetite* – I have joined these two together because exercise increases the amount of serotonin that your brain releases. This hormone is responsible for lifting mood and regulating it, which means you will experience fewer emotional ups and downs, which will help you with battling your binge eating. Also, please note that when you exercise, your appetite and your sleep are better regulated.
- *Protects your brain from stress-related effects* – High levels of stress can detrimentally affect brain function and negatively affect your focus, concentration and

memory. It also increases inflammation within the brain and around the body. Regular exercising will lower your stress levels and improve your brain health.

- *Boosts your confidence levels* – Once you start exercising regularly, you will feel a sense of achievement and accomplishment. That is a great confidence booster.
- *Strengthens your heart* – Giving your heart a good workout regularly strengthens it and reduces the risk factors for cardiovascular issues, including heart attack, cardiovascular disease, and stroke.
- *Boosts your immune system* – Regular exercise boosts your immune system and makes it less likely to be prone to catching a cold. You will feel much stronger inside your body, which improves your mood and confidence levels.

This is not an exhaustive list. Exercise has countless benefits. But the benefits I mentioned are pertinent to your battle with binge eating. The most significant plus point is not just a strengthening of your health, but a focus on improved mood. Feeling happier, more energised, and upbeat can turn your attention from food and bingeing.

How Much Exercise Should You Have?

The bottom line is that any exercise is better than no exercise, so try to focus on moving your body and finding ways to avoid spending too much time sitting. A sedentary lifestyle is one of the leading killers in today's society, and it can negatively affect your physical and mental health.

I already mentioned a few ways of moving your body that are easy to apply in your life and don't take much more time and effort than what you usually spend. Some other ideas are:

- Go for a walk during your lunch break instead of sitting in the office.
- When doing grocery shopping, carry a basket instead of pushing a trolley.
- Do some stretching exercises while waiting for the kettle to boil.
- March on the spot while brushing your teeth.

Anything that allows you to get up and move around more will be beneficial to you. Any movement you do contributes towards getting more exercise.

However, you do need to take on some aerobic exercise too. That means getting your heart rate up, being a little out of breath, and sweat a little. To what level, you may ask.

You need to be active daily. In addition to this, you should do around 2.5 hours of moderate-intensity exercise per week or 75 minutes of high-intensity exercise. Moderate-intensity exercise will get your heart rate up while you can still hold a conversation. On the other hand, high-intensity training is much faster, to the point where you cannot hold a conversation. When doing any workout, listen to your body and don't push yourself too far, especially if you haven't exercised for a while or are in pain.

Strengthening exercises are important too. They can help you work on your legs, back, hips, chest, shoulders and arms. Focus on these types of exercises around two times per week on separate days. You can use the gym for this, but you can also do exercises at home that can bring massive benefits to your body. My book *Get Fit and Healthy in Your Own Home in 20 Minutes or Less* offers an essential daily exercise plan that you can do in the comfort of your home. You can find this book on Amazon.

If you have any health issues, i.e., back problems, knee problems, heart problems, or you're pregnant, make sure that you visit your doctor and get advice for your particular situation.

How to Make Exercise More Fun

Believe it or not, exercise can be great fun!

Exercise needs to be a regular part of your life, and therefore you need to enjoy it. It all comes down to finding an activity that you enjoy and that you want to do. This will help you to stick to it and feel good about doing it.

Think about all the things you enjoy doing and see if you can find an exercise that naturally fits in. For instance, if you love being outdoors, you could go walking regularly and then try and work up to jogging. Did you know that even taking the dog out for a brisk walk counts as exercise? If you love the water, naturally you should try swimming as your exercise of choice. If you like to watch a particular sport on TV, why not joining a team and learning how to play it? Or, if you love dancing, you could join a Zumba class. People with a vast range of different ability levels attend classes at local sports centres and gyms, and new attendees are always welcomed.

Don't be afraid to try something new. You can never know what you might enjoy unless you give it a go. You might think of going to the gym as being painfully boring, but it can be a very sociable and fun place for you to visit regularly. Why not book in for a taster session and see if you like the feel of it?

To add a social aspect to your exercise regime, why not ask a friend to join you during your workouts? By doing this, you are holding yourself accountable. You will not want to cancel an exercise session with your friend because of the commitment you made to them.

Exercise needs to be a regular part of your life, and you need to want to do it and look forward to doing it.

If you have not exercised regularly, make sure you don't push yourself too hard and too fast. You might hurt yourself. Instead, watch your body getting stronger.

I suggest you start exercising slowly, whether walking, jogging, swimming, dancing, etc. and pay attention to how you feel. Try building it up to 15 minutes a day, and then 20 minutes, then 25 minutes, slowly working up until you reach a point that you feel comfortable enough to stick to.

Remember, exercising can help your physical and mental health, and therefore, it can also help you kick binge eating out of your life for good. There is no downside to exercise, provided you don't push it to extremes. Learning to move your body more can increase your energy levels, improve your self-esteem and build confidence.

Chapter Task — How Much Activity are You Getting?

Whilst exercise might seem exhausting, especially if you have not done much of it for a while, start slowly, and you will see that it can be enjoyable and fun all at the same time.

For this chapter task, do the following:

- Think about the amount of exercise you get on a daily and weekly basis. This will give you an idea of how much work you need to do and where you should start.
- Write down on the worksheet any deliberate exercise you took in the last week.
- Add other forms of movement that you did not explicitly think of as exercise (e.g., walking the dog, cleaning the house, playing with your kids).

- Think about both of those categories: deliberate and non-deliberate exercise, and ask yourself: Where can I improve? What can I increase? What can I add?
- If you don't currently exercise, commit to trying a new activity — perhaps you could join a tennis club. You may find that your choice is not right for you, which is OK. Try different things until you find an activity that you like.
- Look for places you could get more activity, such as walking up the stairs at work. And most importantly — commit to doing it daily.
- Just as you did with your food diary, log your exercise and mood in the *Exercise and Mood Diary,* which you will find in the workbook. Start logging the amount of your physical activity into your daily log in the form of minutes and hours, creating a total at the end of the week. Don't forget to pay attention to how exercise makes you feel!

Chapter 9

The Power of Mindfulness: Learn to Recognise True Hunger

"The best way to capture moments is to pay attention. This is how we cultivate mindfulness."

John Kabat-Zinn

Learning to stop binge eating is more than living a healthy life and understanding the problems beneath the surface. It is about discovering and learning tools to help you focus throughout life in general.

Once you identify why you are binge eating, the problem will not magically disappear. You need to work hard to minimise its effect on your life, and you need to focus on creating a healthier environment through diet, exercise, and self-care. But it does not end there either.

It is important to learn different ways to help you overcome any future temptations. Life has many ups and downs. From time to time, the world throws you a curveball, and you need to be able to cope with it in a healthy way, learning how to avoid falling back into old patterns.

In this chapter, you will discover a concept that could help you learn to overcome binge eating by following a few simple principles. It might sound challenging and in-depth but bear with it because it will be effortless to implement once you get into it.

What I am talking about here is mindfulness.

I mentioned it earlier as a useful tactic for combating binge eating, but I didn't go into much detail. This chapter delves more deeply into the benefits of mindfulness, what it can do for you, and how it can help you break binge eating habits, now and in the future.

I am not saying that avoiding binge eating will be an easy task for the rest of your life. As I have already mentioned, sometimes life throws an event at you, which challenges your perception of the situation and makes you want to cling to something familiar. As things currently stand, you may be using binge eating as a way to cope with your feelings and troubles as they arise. This is your default setting — something you may feel the need to fall back into in the future.

What we need to do now is give you another default, something that you can use when things get tough. Something that can prevent you from falling back to your old habits and ruining all the hard work you have done to get over bingeing.

Mindfulness can give you that. It is one of the methods that prove to be very efficient when it comes to behavioural change.

What Is Mindfulness?

Mindfulness is the ability to be in the moment, being aware of what is happening, what you are feeling, and what is going on around you at any given moment.

You might think that you are always aware of what is happening around you, but... are you really? Think about it.

Take a step back and ask yourself how present you are in this moment.

Do you often spend time on your phone, checking your social media messages, watching TV while eating, or texting when you should be talking to your friends or family members? Most of us are guilty of it, and it can rob us of the beauty of the moment we live in.

Mindfulness is more than just being present in the moment. It is about observing situations as they pass you by, rather than feeling the need to react to them as they happen.

For instance, a person who practices mindfulness regularly is often able to side-step unwise reactions because they do not feel the need to act there and then. Instead, they let the situation happen. They let it be, without feeling the need to react, judge, or focus too much on the negative. That doesn't mean they are not paying attention to what is going on around them, it simply means that they take a step back and assess the situation, rather than allowing emotions to rise and control their behaviours.

Mindfulness helps you listen to your body and, as a result, notice changes and allow feelings to be.

Shortly, we are going to look at how awareness and understanding your feelings can help you stop binge eating. This is vital for your overall emotional well-being and a useful way of preventing yourself from reacting adversely in the moment, e.g., resorting to binge eating when a particular emotion comes your way, or lashing out verbally when you become angry.

When you practice mindfulness, you become healthier and happier because you feel more in control. Your emotions are not constantly taking you over and you are not always lamenting about what you did or did not do.

Mindfulness meditation is a perfect way to start your journey. You can practice mindfulness meditation even while you are walking.

I want to encourage you to try the following:

Head out for a walk and make sure your phone is left in your bag or on silent to ensure zero distractions.

- Take a deep breath in through your nose, wait for a second or two, and then exhale slowly out of your mouth, clearing your mind.
- When you are ready, take a look around and choose something from your surroundings. For instance, the tree.
- Focus on the small details, such as green leaves, the sun shining through the branches, or the thick and sturdy trunk. Try to zone in and notice one or more small details.
- By doing this, you are focusing your mind and calming your internal chatter too.
- Then, move on to something else, such as the clouds in the sky.
- Repeat for the duration of your walk.

The idea is that you are not on your phone checking out news and videos of dancing cats. You are not worrying about what will happen tomorrow, or thinking back over something that happened last week. You are in the moment, and you are noticing and focusing on the small details. That is what mindfulness is.

The more often you do this, the easier it will become, and you will also find it much easier to clear your mind while you are doing it. At first, you may find it hard to clear your mind of intrusive thoughts, which are likely to keep flitting in and out. If this happens, allow your thoughts to enter and float away, paying no attention to them.

Give it a go and see how you get on, but remember to persevere. This type of meditation doesn't come easily to most people but the more you do it, the more you will be able to focus for a little longer and then a little longer still. As time goes by, you will also find it easier to stay in the present moment, rather than jumping back to the past or forwards to the future. Remember, the present is the time you live in, and it is the only time you can control.

Mindfulness meditation brings your consciousness into the now and helps you leave the past behind and the future ahead of you.

Allowing yourself to be affected by past failures or fears about the future, can be very disempowering. Focus on what you can control. Do not let your disappointment about the past or anxiety about the future stop you from living your best life. Remember, you live in the now.

Do You Remember What True Hunger Feels Like?

When you binge eat, it is rarely because you are hungry. You might feel peckish, but you often go overboard and don't stop until you are overfull.

When you binge eat, you are not listening to your brain or your stomach. You lose control and do things on auto-pilot.

During the binge eating episode, your mind is not engaged with the present moment. Your focus is on the food (often unhealthy foods), which you believe you need in that instant, only to realise shortly afterwards that food cannot give you what you're looking for.

Mindfulness can help with binge eating avoidance. It keeps you firmly in the here and now, and you are more conscious of your feelings and what they are trying to tell you. You can ask yourself if you are hungry, and you will know for sure. When you have had enough you will notice the feeling of fullness.

If you are under pressure or feel stressed, your body will produce more of the stress hormone cortisol. The body is a finely tuned machine, and when one particular hormone is out of whack, the others are not far behind. Two specific hormones associated with appetite and fullness are called ghrelin and leptin.

Ghrelin tells you that you are hungry, and when you have higher levels of ghrelin, your appetite is stimulated and you will want to eat more. On the other hand, leptin is the hormone that tells you to stop eating because you are full. When you are stressed and cortisol is in control, you will likely have more ghrelin and less leptin. As a result, you want to eat more and you cannot tell when you are full.

So, you might not actually be completely aware of what real hunger feels like. You might have become desensitised to it through your binge eating, depending upon how serious your situation is.

By practising mindfulness, you can be more aware of whether you are hungry, but, more importantly, mindfulness has been shown to lower stress levels. That means that when cortisol levels return to a semblance of normal, your other associated hormones, should too – namely ghrelin. This will reduce the feeling of fake hunger, i.e., when it is just a hormonal reaction and not your actual stomach saying "Hey, I am empty. Feed me!"

What is Mindful Eating, and How can it Help You Avoid Binge Eating?

Mindful eating is the type of mindfulness that will allow you to avoid binge eating and focus on a healthier lifestyle. However, embracing mindfulness will give you the tools to deal with difficult emotions when they arise and avoid acting in ways that might lead you towards bingeing.

Many studies have shown that mindfulness meditation and mindful eating can reduce binge eating and emotional eating[8]. By focusing on eating mindfully, you will also learn to enjoy the food you are eating rather than simply eating for the sake of it. Learning how to chew slowly and enjoy the tastes of your meals and snacks is a great way to appreciate food. When you binge on food, you don't feel the texture or taste the flavours. And you don't feel any enjoyment either.

Mindful eating helps you to engage with food and turn your attention to your eating. When you sit down for a meal, savour the moment. Eat slowly and focus on how your body feels when you eat. By doing this, you can recognise feelings of fullness far easier than if you were eating quickly and mindlessly.

Did you know that it takes around 20 minutes for your brain to recognise that your body is full? That means that by eating quickly, you are not giving yourself 20 minutes to experience satiety. As a result, you eat much more than you would, increasing the chances of digestive problems and weight gain over time. When bingeing on a regular basis and eating fast, you may have forgotten what it feels like to be full and to stop eating due to that feeling.

Mindful eating will allow you to recognise it so you can stop eating whenever you notice the sensation. This makes stopping eating an intentional act, something you are mindful of. It becomes a decision that you made. This gives you a sense of control and, over time, improves your relationship with food. You begin to control your food instead of allowing food to control you.

To begin mindful eating, simply follow these steps:

- *Ask yourself why you are eating* – Before you sit down for a meal, ask yourself whether you are truly hungry, or just thirsty. Checking in with yourself can sometimes be enough to stop you from eating when you are not even hungry, and if you are about to binge, it might be enough to stop you from doing it.

- *Ask yourself if what you are eating is healthy* – It's easy to grab an unhealthy piece of food simply because it is more convenient. One of the ways to stop binge eating is to focus on overall health. Give yourself a moment before you begin eating to ask yourself how healthy the food you are about to eat is. That brief interlude could be enough to stop you from eating something that you may regret later.

- *Notice your emotions while you are eating* – Before you start eating and while you are doing it, be aware of how you feel emotionally. Are you happy that you are enjoying your favourite food? Do you feel nervous or anxious about what you are eating? If so, note it down, and explore the reasons for these feelings afterwards. Once you have stopped eating, it is a good idea to ask yourself how you are feeling. Answers to these questions will help you understand what type of relationship you have with food.

- *Be thankful for the food you are about to eat* – Some people say prayers before eating and thank God for the food they have on the table. You don't need to do this if that is not your thing. You can simply appreciate the food. Be thankful to it for nourishing your body and keeping you healthy.

- *If you feel negative about what you are about to eat in any way, question it* – A significant step towards a binge-free life is to force yourself to pause for a second and ask yourself how you feel about the food you are about to eat. Do you feel guilty? Anxious? Recognise those emotions as negative and learn to see them as triggers. By doing so, it may be enough to snap your mind back into the moment and avoid a bingeing session.

- *Scan your body and ask if you are hungry* – Before you eat, turn your attention to your stomach and look for signs of hunger. Ask yourself if what you are feeling is hunger or another feeling that overwhelms you.

- *Chew slowly and notice the sensations* – When you eat, chew slowly and notice how the food feels in your mouth. Explore the sensations and textures and, before you place the food in your mouth, notice the smell and appearance of the food.

- *Eat in a quiet environment* – It is best to eat in silence if you can. It will give you more chance to relish what you are eating and enjoy the experience. Make sure that you turn off the TV, don't have your phone next to you, and don't read a book or a magazine while you are eating. These distractions will take your mind away from the process and you are likely to start eating mindlessly.

- *Listen to your body while you are eating* – Listen to how your body feels while you are eating and be mindful of whether you are full or nearly full. This will become easier to recognise as you practice, but when your stomach starts to feel full, force yourself to stop

111

eating and be thankful for the food you have eaten. Move away from the table so that you are not tempted to keep picking at any leftovers on your plate.

By using these mindful eating techniques, you can learn to be aware of food and its effects, as well as how it makes you feel. This will give you the strength to deal with any impending binge sessions and allow you to pause, take a moment to breathe, and avoid it happening altogether. Remember, you cannot simply stop binge eating by clicking your fingers and expecting it not to happen again; you need to acquire tools to overcome temptation while identifying and dealing with the root cause.

It is possible to begin mindful eating simply by following the steps above and practising them, but if you think you need a more structured approach, do not hesitate to contact me and book a complimentary call with me to look at your situation and find the best way forward. Together, we will create a plan for you that is realistic and easy to follow. Please go to www.silvanahealthandnutrition.com/booking/ and book your free call at the most convenient time for you. It will be my pleasure to help.

The Huge Benefits of Mindfulness in General

While there is no doubt that mindfulness can help you become more focused on your eating habits and improve your relationship with food, it could also stop you from binge eating too. There is a range of other benefits to look forward to as well. Some of them include:

- Helps you to stay present
- Allows you to savour the small moments in life, without them passing by unnoticed
- Helps you to become completely engaged with what you are doing, therefore learning from it and discovering new solutions and enjoyable activities
- Helps you to deal with problematic situations and emotions as they arrive, without feeling the need to react quickly and without thought
- Gives you less chance to worry about the past and indulge in "what if" and "maybe"
- Gives you less chance to worry about the future and stops you from becoming paralysed by the fear of what is to come, or trying to plan for it too rigidly. The key here is to simply plan for what you need and allow it to flow naturally
- Teaches you how to accept yourself as you are
- Increases happiness levels
- Gives you a greater ability to connect with other people on a deeper level, therefore enhancing relationships and friendships
- Helps relieve stress
- May treat heart disease, but certainly reduces risk factors for cardiovascular problems
- Lowers blood pressure

- Reduces pain in chronic pain conditions, such as arthritis, fibromyalgia, etc.
- Helps you to get a better night's sleep
- Helps to soothe some gastrointestinal issues, such as IBS
- Helps with mental health, i.e. reducing anxiety, depression, and obsessive-compulsive disorder (OCD)
- Can be used as part of a treatment method for substance abuse patients and those with eating disorders

As you can see, there are a lot of positives when it comes to practising mindfulness, so even if you are not doing it with the idea of binge eating reduction in mind, it still brings a huge host of benefits. Yes, it takes time to master it, but it is time well spent.

Chapter Task – Try Mindful Eating

This chapter was about mindful eating and how it can help you to appreciate food more.

Your task is to incorporate mindful eating into your everyday life. If you have never done it before, this could seem overwhelming, but when you do it right, you will be able to experience all the benefits that mindfulness can bring into your life, and with practice, you will be able to master it.

This is your task for this chapter:

- Choose one meal that you know you can eat alone so you can focus.
- Sit at the table in a room free from distractions.
- Concentrate on the food and how it's making you feel. Enjoy it!
- Stop eating when you're full and remove the plate.
- Note how you feel and how this is different from, for example, eating in front of the TV.

Chapter 10

You are Not on Your Own: The Value of a Support Network

"When a person is down in the world, an ounce of help is better than a pound of preaching."

Edward Bulwer-Lytton

It is easy to assume that binge eating is something you should deal with on your own. There is a certain amount of shame and confusion attached to it for the person involved, making it easy for people to hide away and pretend it is not happening. The problem is, when you do that, it compounds everything and makes the situation worse.

In this final chapter, I want to discuss the importance of seeking help and reaching out to your nearest and dearest. I completely understand that you might find it hard to talk to your family and friends about your issues because of fear of judgment. This might stop you from disclosing your feelings.

Casting aside these worries and asking for help is the most essential step towards recovery, and it is also the bravest.

Whatever causes your binge eating, whether you have a diagnosable BED or not, this is something that needs to be addressed. Doing it alone is not impossible, but it can be challenging indeed. You will have more chances to succeed and maintain good results if you have a support network around you.

The Importance of a Support Network

Having a support network when facing a problem can make life infinitely easier. However, when you have a binge eating problem, the most natural thing in the world is to hide your behaviour and to withdraw. This can result in feeling isolated and can create an even bigger problem.

Studies have shown that having good social support can help to reduce the severity and frequency of binge eating[9]. People around you can hold you accountable and steer you away from falling back into old patterns of behaviour.

We all need a support network to help us get through hard times when life gets tough. And in order to be open with someone about your emotions, instead of turning to food, you need to identify people who can be part of your support network.

It's not necessary to have a large circle of people to give you support when you need it. Having only one or two friends can be more than enough. But if you are someone who would prefer to go down the third-party route and find support from people you have never met before, then support groups could be ideal for you. This will allow you to connect with other people who are facing the challenge of binge eating. These groups also have professionals in the field to offer you support.

You can use these groups as a shoulder to cry on when things get hard. It is a resource that you have in your toolkit in case you need it. And it is an extremely valuable one to have.

Understanding where your binge eating is coming from and being open about it is not easy, but it is a brave first step to take. It allows you to deal with difficult times and emotions in a much healthier way.

Your binge eating, as already discussed, has very little to do with physical hunger. It is caused by the way you feel about yourself or your situation. Essentially, your binge eating struggles are a reflection of your life struggles.

The main benefit of a support network is to have someone by your side if you need them. Your support network could be someone who offers you wise words to stop you from moving towards bingeing when your triggers are activated. They will give you support when you feel like things are spiralling out of control, so you can regain control and stop yourself from falling back and bingeing again.

They can also help you build confidence and focus on the positives rather than the negatives. Having the right support can reduce your stress levels and diminish the need for emotional eating. As you can see, the support you get from your network might help you in many different ways.

Do Not Underestimate the Power of Sharing Your Troubles

The first few chapters of this book focused on helping you to learn about your most prevalent reasons for binge eating. In those early stages, I also asked you to do chapter tasks to help you understand why you allow food to control you.

My advice to you is to start sharing your troubles. Your ability to open up about your problems will bring you clarity and put things into perspective so that you can look at the situation from a different angle.

I suggest you find someone who you can trust to share your problems with. It could be anyone — a qualified counsellor or a close friend. Those are the people who will not judge you. They will understand you and be there when you need their support. Be open and honest with them.

It's also important to be willing to listen to yourself and make sure that you always pay attention to your needs. Learning how to talk about your needs in a caring manner and offering yourself comfort without indulging in foods is crucial. And if you don't know how to comfort yourself, then you must learn how to ask others for what you need. Whether you need love or attention, I can guarantee that you will not find it inside food. And the more you binge, the more you will push away what you really need.

Be open with your support network and with yourself. Only then will you understand the connection between the way you feel and the way you eat. And only then will you realise that your binge eating will never provide the solution to your problems.

The Benefits of Support Groups and Where to Find Them

There are support groups out there for every possible problem, including binge eating. There are many people in the same situation as you, and each one of them needs support, just like you. Therefore, it makes sense to create support groups and come together with one thing in common — the very thing that causes them discomfort and upset.

The hardest part about accessing support groups is finding the right one for you. You have two options here. The first is to look online and to join a virtual support group. There are many Facebook groups, and I am sure you will find a group that meets your needs quite easily. When you join the group, make sure that you actively participate because that way, you are creating the connections I talked about earlier.

You could also find an in-person support group if that makes you more comfortable. In many ways, this is a better option for meeting people and finding new friends in your local area. These groups often meet weekly, and these face-to-face meetings typically take place in health centres or community centres. Again, in these groups, you don't have to speak if you don't want to, but you will be encouraged to do so. Sharing is an excellent route towards success, so it's important to participate rather than restricting yourself to listening on the sidelines.

The more energy and effort you put into interacting with other members of your chosen support group, the more you will get out of it.

The benefits are pretty straightforward. Support groups are made of people who have the same problem as you. That means you are among like-minded people who understand what you're going through, which can be very valuable in making you feel less alone in your struggles with food.

It could be that your particular area does not have any support groups, in which case, online support could be the best route for you. The Internet may have many downsides, but it is a fantastic invention in terms of reaching out to people and connecting.

Regarding where to find support groups, I suggest that you check social media pages and see if you can find advertisements or groups in your local area. You can also look on the notice boards at your doctor's surgery, library, or the local community centre. Church halls are another potential location for support groups to meet, so look for flyers on noticeboards there.

If you find nothing from your search, the next best thing is to ask your doctor, who will undoubtedly have a list of resources you can tap into. Even if these are not local, there will always be an online route to look into.

When to Seek Help from Your Doctor

Binge eating incorporates a broad spectrum of behaviours, from someone who binges infrequently to someone who has a full-blown BED. Overeating now and then, such as over Christmas, on birthdays, or during other special occasions, is very normal and is usually done with intent. But overeating large amounts of food frequently and very quickly, and not stopping to taste the food, is a reason for concern.

Many people can overcome their binge eating issues at home with self-help methods and access support from their loved ones or support groups. If you are concerned about your binge eating and feel that it is getting worse, and you cannot handle it anymore or are moving into BED diagnosis territory, it might be a good time to seek help from a professional.

The decision to reach out for formal help is not easy to make, but it might be necessary. Many people falsely believe that psychological problems are a sign of weakness. This could not be further from the truth. Reaching out for help with something that torments you day in and day out, which has been a private battle that not many people know about, shows that you are strong for admitting that you need support with your issues. It is also the right thing to do.

If you have reached this point, I want to congratulate you for recognising your own needs and prioritising them — pat yourself on the back for doing that.

There are a few management options for binge eating when it reaches the point where you feel you cannot manage it yourself. I will outline those in the next section, but I would like to invite you once again to book your complimentary call with me. In that call, we will talk about your issues, and together, we will explore the best ways for you to overcome them.

To book your complimentary call with me, please visit silvanahealthandnutrition.com/booking. It will be a real pleasure to help you and work with you through a recovery plan in detail. From there, I can assist you in different ways. Receiving support from a professional person in these situations can make a world of difference.

Potential Management Options for Binge Eating

There are a few management options for binge eating. They delve into the deeper reasons behind the impulse to binge and are intended to help you develop coping strategies. These are not for everyone, and it depends on how you feel, what you want to try, and what your doctor feels is the best fit for you.

There are four main management options that you might be offered:

- Cognitive behaviour therapy (CBT)
- Interpersonal psychotherapy
- Dialectical behavioural therapy
- Behavioural weight loss therapy

All of these management options work to unearth the more profound meaning of your bingeing and identify patterns. Cognitive behaviour therapy, known as CBT more commonly, is most likely to be the first option offered to you. This type of treatment explores the connections between your emotions and eating patterns. By identifying triggers and avoiding them or confronting them, you will be able to put into place strategies to help you avoid bingeing.

Interpersonal psychotherapy is a very intense management programme that usually takes place over 12-16 weeks. This therapy focuses on solving any interpersonal problems you may have and discovering their connection with your symptoms. Once you are aware of your symptoms, you can then put into place strategies to deal with your issues.

Dialectical behaviour therapy, or DBT, is another type of treatment used for various conditions. Just like CBT, it has more than one use. Still, it is often used to treat mood problems, borderline personality disorder and to identify and change patterns of behaviour, especially in people who regularly self-harm or use a particular substance, or, in this case, turn to food to deal with problems.

Finally, behavioural weight loss therapy might be very beneficial for someone who binge eats and has a weight issue alongside it. This is a programme that is typically delivered over a few months, (usually six months) and focuses on health, diet, exercise, and changing negative behaviours. The therapy is delivered via sessions and lifestyle alterations.

One size does not fit all. That is the most important thing to remember when learning about management techniques.

It is also important to understand that you might never be 100% cured of binge eating. The impulse to binge might always be present; however, it is in your power to turn the volume down to the point where you do not hear it — put it on mute, if you will. Then, over time, you learn coping strategies that keep it on silent so that you never have to hear it again.

That does not mean that you are not going to have an occasional urge. It simply means that when you do, you will know how to manage it, since you will be familiar with the techniques to use to side-step a potential pitfall, which will stop you from falling foul of binge eating.

For many people, whether they work through a therapy programme or try to handle their binge eating behaviour via talking to someone about their issues and making lifestyle changes, the biggest problem they experience is dealing with accidental slip-ups. When something happens, perhaps a negative event, or receiving bad news, they forget everything they learnt and go back to their old habits and start bingeing again. They assume that they have failed because of one slip-up, and therefore there is no point in trying again.

This kind of mindset is not going to help you overcome your problems. If you slip up, I suggest you stand up, dust yourself off, and then try again. Failure is good. Do not be disappointed when things do not go well. Accepting failures is an integral part of life. It helps you to focus your energy on doing better next time.

Remember, you are on a journey and not a one-day event. You will inevitably face many ups and downs on the road. If you allow yourself to have occasional slip-ups, you will never feel like you have failed. Failing is a belief and not concrete evidence.

On your good days — when things go well, be proud of yourself for doing your best. And on your bad days — when things do not go too well, be proud of yourself for trying to do your best.

Chapter Task — Ask for Help

This chapter has focused on the importance of support and reaching out for help if you feel you need it. For many people, admitting a problem can be difficult, but it is the most crucial step towards progress.

Your final chapter task is to be brave, reach out, and ask for help.

You cannot take on the world alone and win. You cannot expect to work your way through hardships and never stumble. Give yourself a break and pat yourself on the back for simply being the person you are. And if you feel you need help and support, listen to that need and do what it tells you. Allowing yourself to be open about your problems and permitting yourself to feel vulnerable shows how strong you are.

Asking for help puts you in a strong position. It shows you are courageous and know how to take care of yourself. It means you are not neglecting your needs but giving yourself a chance to connect to your worth.

Conclusion

Congratulations on reading this book to the end! You have shown the determination you need to defeat your binge eating and create a healthy relationship with food.

As you have seen, binge eating is a common issue, but it can be extremely dangerous over the long-term. Whether or not you have been diagnosed with BED, using such a damaging method for handling your emotional state will not serve you well, either mentally or physically.

Throughout this book, I have given you actionable steps and advice to follow. You have learned what binge eating disorder (BED) is, what factors can cause it, and how to identify it. As you have seen, BED should not be confused with occasional overeating. There are clear signs to help you recognise whether your eating habits are associated with a binge eating disorder. The exercises at the end of each chapter can help you recognise the danger signs and equip you with the knowledge of how to tackle them

If you completed tasks at the end of each chapter, you should be able to clearly see how they link to one another, creating a method of overcoming binge eating in a slow and sure manner. If you have not yet done the tasks, you have a chance to do them now.

I want to remind you that you can download the workbook with all the tasks in one place at bit.ly/binge-eating-workbook. I suggest you work through each task slowly, ensuring you complete them thoroughly and commit yourself to the task at hand.

Be honest with yourself about what it means to you to overcome your binge eating. If it is high on your priority list, then treat it that way, and work towards fulfilling your need. If you distort the truth or hold anything back, the only person you are cheating is yourself.

Binge eating is not something to take lightly. It is not just eating a bit too much occasionally or liking chocolate a little too much. It is an emotional reaction that turns into action, which will damage your health over the long-term if you ignore it. You could be reading this thinking that you are not at a place where you have a diagnosable BED. I want to point out that it doesn't mean that the advice throughout this book is not relevant to you or that your situation is not as dangerous.

In this book, you were equipped with the knowledge about developing strategies and ensuring that you eat regular, balanced meals to get your eating under control and overcome bingeing. Emphasis was also placed on the importance of being physically active and practising mindfulness.

As you have seen, binge eating is not just about food. The food is simply the coping mechanism for the underlying issues. In the same way, fighting BED is not only about controlling your food intake.

This book showed you how to dig deeper and explore the reasons for your unhealthy eating habits to help you to unlock your future potential.

It is vital to remember that the fight against BED is a long-term process. It is not something you are going to crack in a week. The habits and systems you set up in the chapter tasks will equip you to replace the old, self-destructive behaviours with positive ones, but you must follow those processes.

Binge eating can be a difficult, disheartening struggle, especially if you try to hide it from others.

As I explained in the final chapter of this book, it is very easy to slip back into your old habits. Therefore, it is advisable to have support in your struggle against BED. This could be a friend or relative, or you might join a support group. And if you want more structured support centred on your personal needs, I can offer just that.

Why me?

Besides my training and experience in psychology, counselling, and nutrition, and working with clients for many years, I have experienced the impact of changing my own diet and lifestyle. I know many of the struggles you are going through — but I am also aware of the amazing results you will experience if you stick with it. I can be with you every step of the way to guarantee your success.

What next?

If you are going to beat binge eating, you need to do this:

- Complete all the tasks in this book — and then redo them.
- Develop plans to eat healthily and reduce the cravings that lead to binge eating.
- Start being physically active. This will improve both your general health and your emotional health.
- Practice mindfulness to control your mental state and avoid reactive behaviour leading to unhealthy habits.
- Build yourself a support network to help you get through the hard times.
- Book a call with me to explore the reasons behind your unhealthy eating patterns.

Defeating a binge eating disorder will not be a breeze, but you can do it with determination and the right tools. This book has given you the tools you need, and the determination is already within you. You just need to access it.

All that is left now is for me to wish you the most extraordinary luck in the world. Please reach out for your complimentary consultation with me, as mentioned earlier in the book.

Simply head to www.silvanahealthandnutrition.com/booking and follow the instructions to book your slot.

You now have all the tools you need to start your journey towards a binge-free future. Make it a priority, and use your toolbox full of tools to kick binge eating out of your life for good. If you need my help, I am here. Reach out!

If you enjoyed this book and found it helpful, please go to http://viewbook.at/breakthebinge and leave a review on Amazon. By doing that, we can reach out to more people and help them to start a binge-free life.

Lots of love xx

Silvana

About the Author

Having spent over 20 years working with people experiencing a range of health issues, Silvana Siskov has expanded her reach to help people via print. "Break the Binge Eating Cycle" is the latest in the range of books she has published and focuses on helping people with specific health concerns, both physically and mentally.

Working within the niches of mental health, eating disorders, and weight management, to name just a few, Silvana's main areas of expertise include giving sound and practical advice that focuses upon emotional support first and foremost.

Having changed her lifestyle for the better, Silvana is more than aware of the critical role of health and well-being in all aspects of people's lives, giving her practical and personal experience to fall back on when advising her clients. As a result, she is able to guide them in the right direction, giving them help and support in the areas they need the most.

With her years of experience, Silvana can connect with her clients and advise them to make the changes they need to feel empowered and move towards a brighter and healthier future.

She finds true pleasure in supporting her clients and working closely with them on a one-on-one basis. She extends her work into the community, with talks and workshops for those who prefer a more sociable atmosphere. Silvana understands that to get the best out of people, she needs to help them from the inside, so they can flourish on the outside. She supports their emotional and psychological needs and encourages them to lead a healthy lifestyle.

Silvana's overall mission is to empower and motivate people, helping them to create a deeper connection to themselves. By doing so, they can achieve whatever they put their minds to, living their very best lives.

Referenced Studies

Throughout this book, the following studies have been referenced:

1. Ekern, J. (2018). "Am I Overeating or Do I Have a Binge Eating Disorder" https://www.eatingdisorderhope.com/information/binge-eating-disorder/binge-eating-disorder-vs-basic-overeating-what-is-the-difference
2. Polivy, J., Coleman, J., and Herman, C. P. (2005). The effect of deprivation on food cravings and eating behaviour in restrained and unrestrained eaters. PubMed. https://pubmed.ncbi.nlm.nih.gov/16261600/
3. Stice, E., Davis, K., Miller, N. P., and Marti, C. N. (2008). Fasting Increases Risk for Onset of Binge Eating and Bulimic Pathology: A 5-Year Prospective Study. NCBI. https://www.ncbi.nlm.nih.gov/pmc/articles/PMC2850570/
4. Weigle, D. S., Breen, P. A., Matthys, C. C., Callahan, H. S., Meeuws, K. E., Burden., V. R., and Purnell, J. Q. (2005). A high-protein diet induces sustained

reductions in appetite, ad libitum caloric intake, and body weight despite compensatory changes in diurnal plasma leptin and ghrelin concentrations. PubMed.

https://pubmed.ncbi.nlm.nih.gov/16002798/

5. Walleghen, E. L., Orr, J. S., Gentile, C. L., and Davy, B. M. (2007) Pre-meal water consumption reduces meal energy intake in older but not younger subjects. PubMed.

https://pubmed.ncbi.nlm.nih.gov/17228036/

6. Levine, M. D., Marcus, M. D., and Moulton, P. (1996). Exercise in the treatment of binge eating disorder. PubMed.

https://pubmed.ncbi.nlm.nih.gov/8932555/

7. Pendleton, V. R., Goodrick, G. K., Walke, S., Poston, C., Reeves, R. S., and Foreyt, J. P. (2002). Exercise augments the effects of cognitive-behavioural therapy in the treatment of binge eating. PubMed.

https://pubmed.ncbi.nlm.nih.gov/11920978/

8. Katterman, S. N., Kleinman, B. M., Hood, M. M., Nackers, L. M., and Corsica, J. A. (2014). (n.d.). Mindfulness meditation as an intervention for binge eating, emotional eating, and weight loss: a systematic review. PubMed.

https://pubmed.ncbi.nlm.nih.gov/24854804/

9. Goodrick, G. K., Pendleton, V. R., Kimball, K. T., Walker, S., Poston, C., Reeves, R. S. and Foreyt, J. P. (1999). Binge eating severity, self-concept, dieting self-efficacy and social support during treatment of binge eating disorder. PubMed.

https://pubmed.ncbi.nlm.nih.gov/10441245/

Helpful Resources

Books by Silvana Siskov:

- *"Get Your Sparkle Back: 10 Steps to Weight Loss and Overcoming Emotional Eating."* The book is available on Amazon. Go to http://viewbook.at/sparkle.
- *"Live Healthy on a Tight Schedule: 5 Easy Ways for Busy People to Develop Sustainable Habits Around Food, Exercise and Self-Care."* The book is available on Amazon. Go to http://viewbook.at/livehealthy.
- *"Get Fit and Healthy in Your Own Home in 20 Minutes or Less: An Essential Daily Exercise Plan and Simple Meal Ideas to Lose Weight and Get the Body You Want."* The book is available on Amazon. Go to http://viewbook.at/get-fit.
- *"Get Fit and Healthy on a Tight Schedule 2 Books in 1."* The book is available on Amazon. Go to http://viewbook.at/get-fit2books.
- *"Beat Your Menopause Weight Gain: Balance Hormones, Stop Middle-Age Spread, Boost Your Health And Vitality."* The book is available on Amazon. Go to http://viewbook.at/beat-menopause.

- *"Free Yourself From Hot Flushes and Night Sweats: The Essential Guide to a Happy And Healthy Menopause."* The book is available on Amazon. Go to http://viewbook.at/healthy-menopause.
- *"Manage Your Menopause 2 Books in 1: How to Balance Hormones and Prevent Middle-Age Spread."* The book is available on Amazon. Go to http://viewbook.at/manage-menopause.

Free Mini-Courses:

- *Discover 10 Secrets of Successful Weight Loss*
- *This is How to Start Eating Less Sugar*
- *Learn How to Boost Your Energy – 11 Easy Ways*
- *Your Guide to a Happy and Healthy Menopause*
- *This is How to Lose Weight in Your 40's and Beyond*

Free Courses Available at:

www.silvanahealthandnutrition.com/course/

Made in the USA
Middletown, DE
17 May 2021